Table of Contents

Introduction

- Welcome to the Chaos   p4

Chapter 1: Before Baby: Preparing for a Growing Family p5
  - Prepping the Older Kids for a New Sibling p5
  - Juggling Pregnancy with Toddlers p9
  - Setting Up the Home for Another Baby p13

Chapter 2: Heading to the Hospital p20
  - What to Pack for Delivery Day p20
  - Coordinating Childcare for Your Other Children p25
  - Handling Multiple Births in a Short Time Frame p29

Chapter 3: Being in the Hospital p34
  - Navigating Labor and Delivery p34
  - Hospital Recovery Tips for the Busy Mom p39
  - Introducing the New Baby to Their Siblings p44

Chapter 4: Surviving the Newborn Stage p50
  - Adjusting to Life with a Newborn p50
  - Managing the Needs of Different-Aged Kids p54
  - Bonding with Your Newborn p58

Chapter 5: Breastfeeding and Pumping Essentials p62
  - Managing Breastfeeding with Older Kids Around p62
  - Efficient Pumping to Stay Flexible p67
  - Navigating Supply and Demand with Multiple Little Ones p73

Chapter 6: Sleep Training for Different Ages p80
   - Creating a Routine that Works for All Kids p80
   - Sleep Training Techniques for the Newborn p84
   - Managing Sleep Regressions with Other Toddlers p89

Chapter 7: Teething p94
   -Facts about teething p94
   -Signs and cues of teething p97
   -Soothe your teething baby p100

Chapter 8: Dealing with Rashes p103
   - Common Infant and Toddler Rashes p103
   - Remedies that Worked p112
   - What to Watch for and When to Call the Doctor p118

Chapter 9: Potty Training p122
   - Timing Potty Training p122
   - Training Tips for Busy Parents p127
   - Handling Setbacks   p132

Chapter 10: Meal Planning for a Busy Household p147
  - Simple and Nutritious Meals for the Whole Family p137
  - Feeding Toddlers and a Newborn at the Same Time p142
  - Handling Picky Eaters and Special Diets p148

Chapter 11: Traveling with a Full House p153
  - Packing for All Ages p153
  - Making Travel Fun and Stress-Free p157
  - Tips for Road Trips and Air Travel p161

Chapter 12: Managing Screen Time for Different Ages p166
  - Setting Age-Appropriate Limits p166
  - Earning Screen Time p171
  -Finding Best Apps, Shows, and Games for Young Children p175

Chapter 13: Self-Care for the Overwhelmed Parent p180
  - Finding Moments for Yourself p180
  - Mental Health Tips for Handling Stress p184
  - Balancing Your Needs with Your Family's p189

Chapter 14: Keeping Your Relationship Strong p195
  - Maintaining Connection Amid Parenthood p195
  - Date Nights at Home p201
  - Open Communication Tips p206

Chapter 15: Is Your Family Complete? p212
  - Deciding if You Can Handle Another Baby p212
  - There's No "Right" Time to Have a Baby p217
  - Imagining the Future of Your Family p223
  - Trusting Your Instincts and Vision for Your Family p228

Dedication p233

Welcome to the Chaos

Before the chaos, I didn't think I was ready. Like so many of us, I doubted myself, questioning whether I was good enough, prepared enough, or even capable of handling the challenges ahead. The idea of being a parent—especially with an older stepchild already in the picture—felt overwhelming. But then, as each little one entered my life, I realized that readiness isn't something you have from the start. It's something you grow into.

With each child, I learned, adapted, and somehow became ready. The things that once felt impossible or intimidating turned into lessons that equipped me for the next step. I found that the key to surviving—and thriving—was to take what I learned from each child and use it for the next. This is not to say it was smooth sailing from there; every child brought their own unique challenges, and just when I thought I had it all figured out, I would be thrown a new curveball.

What I discovered along the way was that no matter how much experience I had, every child was different, and the journey was never the same. I was constantly learning and adapting. Some things worked well with one child but didn't with the next. It took a lot of humility and patience to realize that I wasn't failing—I was just continuously growing. What helped me the most was the ability to keep what worked and learn from what didn't. That mindset became my lifeline through the beautiful chaos of raising four kids and balancing the dynamic of having a stepchild.

At the heart of it all, I learned that the most important thing you can bring to parenthood is unconditional love and an open mind. Each child has their own needs, and the best thing we can do as parents is strive to find what works best for them. It's not about perfection or having all the answers from the beginning—it's about learning, adapting, and giving yourself grace along the way.
If you can do that, you'll be okay. Welcome to the chaos—you're more ready than you think.

Chapter 1
Before Baby
Preparing for a Growing Family

Prepping the Older Kids for a New Sibling

Preparing older kids for a new sibling can help ease the transition and make them feel included in the process.

1. Ask Them How They Feel About the New Sibling
  - Why it's important: Understanding their emotions helps you address any concerns or excitement they have. It also reassures them that their feelings matter.

2. Give Them a Role as "Special Helper"
  - Why it's important: Giving them a role in caring for the baby makes them feel responsible and needed, helping prevent jealousy.

3. Get Them a Stuffed Animal to Care For
  - Why it's important: It helps them practice being nurturing by dressing, diapering, and caring for their "baby," which mimics how they'll interact with the new sibling.

4. Record the Baby's Heartbeat and a Loving Message
  - Why it's important: Having a tangible connection to the new baby through a heartbeat recording makes the idea of a sibling more real and personal.

5. Talk Constantly About How They'll Love Each Other
  - Why it's important: Reassurance helps create a positive image of their future bond and sets the stage for a loving relationship between siblings.

6. Discuss the Challenges of a New Baby
   - Why it's important: Preparing them for the reality of crying and constant attention helps manage expectations and reduces frustration when the baby arrives.

7. Encourage Them to Be a Role Model
   - Why it's important: Emphasizing how much the baby will look up to them gives them a sense of pride and motivates them to teach the baby positive behaviors.

8. Talk About the Baby as a "New Best Friend"
   - Why it's important: Framing the baby as someone they can bond with helps build excitement and a sense of connection even before the baby is born.

9. Show Baby Pictures of Themselves
   - Why it's important: Helping them understand they were once babies too makes it easier for them to empathize with the new sibling's needs.

10. Let Them Help Set Up the Baby's Space
   - Why it's important: Including them in preparing the nursery or baby items helps them feel involved and part of the new chapter.

11. Read Books About New Siblings Together
   - Why it's important: Books can introduce the concept of a new sibling in a fun, relatable way, helping them understand the upcoming changes.

12. Explain How Babies Need Extra Attention at First
   - Why it's important: Being honest about the baby's needs reduces confusion when they see you spending a lot of time caring for the newborn.

13. Give Them Special "Big Sibling" Tasks
   - Why it's important: Assigning simple, age-appropriate tasks fosters a sense of accomplishment and makes them feel important in the baby's life.

14. Talk About How They Can Teach the Baby New Things
   - Why it's important: Highlighting how they can teach the baby fun and good behaviors creates excitement and encourages responsibility.

15. Remind Them That They Are Loved
   - Why it's important: Reassuring them of their place in the family prevents feelings of being replaced or left out.

16. Set Aside One-on-One Time With Them
   - Why it's important: Maintaining one-on-one time reassures them that their relationship with you won't change, even with the new sibling.

17. Involve Them in Baby's Care Decisions
   - Why it's important: Letting them help pick out baby clothes or toys allows them to have a say, making them feel included.

18. Talk About How Babies Learn from Older Siblings
   - Why it's important: Highlighting the impact they will have on the baby's development builds a sense of importance and responsibility.

19. Prepare Them for Visitors and Attention the Baby Will Get
   - Why it's important: Explaining that the baby might get a lot of attention from others helps them understand and prevents jealousy.

20. Make Family Time Before the Baby Arrives
   - Why it's important: Spending quality time together before the baby arrives strengthens your bond and reassures them that they are valued in the family.

By taking these steps, you help the older kids feel involved, valued, and ready for the new addition to the family. It's all about keeping them included in the process and maintaining open communication.

When our family was growing, we wanted to make sure our little ones felt included and prepared for the arrival of their new sibling. We found a way to make the anticipation a little sweeter and to help them adjust to the idea of a new baby joining our lives.

For my stepson, who was just five at the time, we gave him something special—a bear with our new baby's heartbeat inside. After the heartbeat, the bear played a sweet message with our voices, telling him how much we loved him. This little bear quickly became his world. He dressed it in diapers and tiny clothes, treating it just like the real baby he was about to meet. At the park, he would bring the bear and gently place it in the baby swing, pushing it with all the tenderness of a big brother practicing his new role. He'd even tuck the bear into a front pack, wearing it proudly as if it were his very own. At night, the bear never left his side; it was his special connection to his soon-to-be sibling, and he loved it with his whole heart. And even now, years later, he still has that bear, a cherished reminder of that time when he first became a big brother.

For our toddler, who was just two, we decided on a baby doll. It became our tool for teaching her how to be gentle, using soft hands and learning how to hold and care for a little one. We spent time showing her how to play nice, guiding her tiny hands to cradle the doll's head and whisper sweet words. She loved wrapping the doll in blankets and pretending to feed it, imitating everything she saw us do, soaking in every lesson about being kind and gentle.

These simple moments, playing with a bear and a baby doll, made such a difference. By the time the new baby arrived, both of them were more than ready. They knew how to be soft, careful, and loving around their new sibling. The bear and the doll had been more than just toys; they were their first steps into their new roles as big brother and big sister, helping them feel included, important, and excited for the new adventure our family was about to begin.

Juggling Pregnancy with Toddlers

Managing pregnancy while caring for a toddler is crucial to maintaining your physical and mental well-being, as balancing both demands helps prevent burnout. It allows you to establish a routine that supports both your toddler's development and your own needs for rest and recovery. By preparing early, you can ease the transition for your toddler and create a smoother adjustment when the new baby arrives.

1. Create a Consistent Sleep Routine
   -Benefits: Helps toddlers feel secure and rested, giving you quiet time to rest and reduce pregnancy fatigue.

2. Involve Toddlers in Talking and Singing to the Baby
   -Benefits: Builds early bonding and helps toddlers adjust to the idea of a sibling while keeping you connected to both.

3. Find a Pregnancy Pillow and Belly Band
   -Benefits: Improves your sleep and comfort, which enhances your patience and energy for engaging with your toddler.

4. Start Transitioning Toddlers Out of Your Room
   -Benefits: Helps your toddler get used to independence while preparing your space for the newborn's arrival.

5. Use a Toddler Carrier or Stroller for Walks
   -Benefits: Promotes exercise for you while keeping the toddler entertained, reducing the need for more active playtime.

6. Set Up a Special Quiet Time Activity Box
   -Benefits: Provides toddlers with solo play opportunities, allowing you moments of rest during the day.

7. Simplify Mealtime with Easy, Nutrient-Rich Foods
   -Benefits: Ensures your toddler is getting proper nutrition while giving you more time to rest and less stress about meal prep.

8. Encourage Independent Play
   -Benefits: Fosters creativity and independence in your toddler while giving you much-needed breaks during the day.

9. Prepare for Fewer Outings as Your Due Date Nears
   -Benefits: Eases the transition for your toddler to a less active lifestyle while reducing your physical strain.

10. Plan Toddler-Friendly Pregnancy Exercises
   -Benefits: Keeps both you and your toddler active in a gentle, safe way, promoting a healthy pregnancy and bonding.

11. Introduce a Simple 'Helper' Role
   -Benefits: Makes toddlers feel involved and useful while lightening some tasks for you, like tidying up toys or fetching items.

12. Practice Baby Care with a Doll
   -Benefits: Helps toddlers understand how to be gentle with the baby, easing their transition to being a sibling.

13. Limit Screen Time and Encourage Hands-On Activities
   -Benefits: Stimulates your toddler's brain while reducing reliance on screen time, keeping their routine enriching while you focus on the pregnancy.

14. Stick to a Calm Evening Routine
   -Benefits: A calming wind-down helps your toddler sleep better, ensuring you both get more rest at night.

15. Find Comfortable Clothing for Yourself
   -Benefits: Staying comfortable allows you to engage with your toddler without discomfort or frustration.

16. Use a Toy Rotation System
   -Benefits: Keeps toys fresh and exciting for your toddler, providing them with focused play while you conserve your energy.

17. Schedule Short, Manageable Playdates
   -Benefits: Helps maintain your toddler's social skills without overwhelming you with long, physically demanding activities.

18. Teach Toddlers to Retrieve Light Items
   -Benefits: Turns toddlers into little helpers while saving you energy, teaching responsibility in a fun way.

19. Designate a Cozy Rest Spot for Yourself Near Play Areas
   -Benefits: Allows you to keep an eye on your toddler while resting comfortably, ensuring you're both in the same space.

20. Focus on Positive Reinforcement and Gentle Boundaries
   -Benefits: Encourages good behavior in your toddler without needing constant discipline, reducing stress for both of you as you prepare for the baby.

Each of these tips helps maintain balance, supporting your toddler's development while considering your energy and comfort during pregnancy.

Juggling pregnancy with a toddler is no easy task. While my body was busy growing a new life, my energetic toddler was constantly on the move, bouncing around with endless energy. It was hard because, at their age, they didn't fully understand what was happening. They were rough, climbing on me when I least expected it, and full of life when I just wanted to rest. Keeping up with them was exhausting, and I quickly learned that the only way to survive was through preparation and routines.

Getting my toddler on a sleep schedule became essential. Those precious moments when they were down for a nap or settled in bed at night gave me the downtime I desperately needed. But it wasn't just about me—my toddler thrived on the consistency of a routine, knowing what to expect each day. It helped them feel secure and calm, and in turn, it made our days a little smoother.

I found that preparation was key. If I set things up the night before—whether it was laying out clothes, prepping snacks, or just getting the diaper bag ready—our mornings were so much easier. Even simple things like planning meals ahead of time made a big difference. It was amazing how these little habits helped keep us on track.

Of course, life doesn't always go according to plan. When we got off our routine, things could go a little crazy. Meltdowns, skipped naps, and chaos would creep in, reminding me just how much kids need that consistency. But I also learned it's okay to be flexible. Life happens, and it's okay to stray from the routine sometimes. What mattered most was that we tried to find our way back, using preparation and routines as our guideposts.

Through it all, I realized that routines weren't just about keeping my toddler in check—they were a way to help us both thrive during this time of transition. And while every day wasn't perfect, sticking to a routine made juggling pregnancy with a toddler just a little bit easier, giving us both the structure we needed in the midst of change.

Setting Up the Home for Another Baby

Getting your home ready for the baby before their arrival helps reduce stress and ensures you have everything you need for a smooth transition. Involving your family, especially your spouse and other children, fosters a sense of teamwork and helps everyone feel prepared for the new addition. It also creates a shared experience that strengthens family bonds while making the home more organized and baby-friendly.

1. Rearrange the Nursery
- What to Do: Organize the space to fit both baby and toddler essentials.
- Money-Saving Option: Use the furniture you already have and repurpose items.
- Benefits: Saves money and time, reduces clutter.
- No-Budget Option: Buy new nursery furniture and storage solutions.
- Benefits: Fresh, organized space tailored to both children's needs.

2. Reuse Older Sibling's Baby Clothes
- What to Do: Sort through the older child's baby clothes for the newborn.
- Money-Saving Option: Reuse hand-me-downs from your first child.
- Benefits: Saves money and reduces waste.
- No-Budget Option: Purchase a new wardrobe for the baby.
- Benefits: New items tailored to your preferences and style.

3. Create a Shared Closet Space
- What to Do: Organize a shared space for toddler and baby clothes.
- Money-Saving Option: Use existing closet organizers and bins.
- Benefits: Makes organizing easier without spending extra money.
- No-Budget Option: Install a custom-built closet system.
- Benefits: Maximizes storage and keeps everything organized.

4. Set Up a Baby Corner in Your Bedroom
- What to Do: Create a safe space for the baby's bassinet and supplies.
- Money-Saving Option: Use a hand-me-down bassinet and existing furniture.
- Benefits: No additional costs, easy to set up.
- No-Budget Option: Purchase a new bassinet and matching furniture.
- Benefits: Stylish, new setup for your bedroom and baby.

5. Install a Second Baby Monitor
- What to Do: Add a monitor to keep an eye on both kids.
- Money-Saving Option: Buy a second-hand or refurbished monitor.
- Benefits: Peace of mind without overspending.
- No-Budget Option: Purchase a top-of-the-line dual baby monitor system.
- Benefits: High-tech monitoring with advanced features like video and audio.

6. DIY or Repurpose Furniture
- What to Do: Refurbish old furniture for the baby.
- Money-Saving Option: Use secondhand furniture and DIY updates.
- Benefits: Cuts down on the cost of buying new items, personalizes the space.
- No-Budget Option: Purchase new, stylish baby furniture.
- Benefits: Fresh, coordinated nursery décor with modern functionality.

7. Prepare a Diaper Changing Station for Each Room
- What to Do: Set up multiple diaper stations around the house.
- Money-Saving Option: Repurpose existing baskets or tables for stations.
- Benefits: Saves on buying extra furniture, maximizes current items.
- No-Budget Option: Buy stylish, matching changing stations for multiple rooms.
- Benefits: Convenient and cohesive setups for easy diaper changes.

8. Declutter and Make Space
- What to Do: Clear out unnecessary items to make room for the baby.
- Money-Saving Option: Declutter for free by donating or selling old items.
- Benefits: Opens up space without spending any money.
- No-Budget Option: Hire a professional organizer.
- Benefits: Expert organization and maximized space efficiency.

9. Choose Dual-Purpose Baby Gear
- What to Do: Find gear that works for both baby and toddler.
- Money-Saving Option: Invest in multifunctional gear like a convertible high chair.
- Benefits: Saves money and space with one item for both children.
- No-Budget Option: Buy separate high-end gear for each child.
- Benefits: Tailored items for each child's needs and preferences.

10. Set Up a Feeding and Pumping Station
- What to Do: Organize a station with all feeding essentials, including a pump, extra bottle rack, mini fridge, bottle warmer, burp rags, diapers, wipes, extra onesies, water for yourself, and a hands-free pumping bra.
- Money-Saving Option: Use a small table or cart you already own, and repurpose containers for organizing essentials.
-Benefits: Easy access to all feeding tools in one place, saving time and effort. Staying hydrated with water nearby also helps with milk production.
- No-Budget Option: Purchase a new, stylish furniture piece for the station and invest in high-quality feeding equipment, including a top-tier pump, fridge, and bottle warmer.
- Benefits: A sleek, organized, and efficient setup for feeding and pumping, making the process smoother and more comfortable.

11. Prepare Hand-Me-Down Toys
- What to Do: Use older sibling's toys for the baby.
- Money-Saving Option: Repurpose toddler's old toys.
- Benefits: Saves money and creates a sense of sharing for the older child.
- No-Budget Option: Buy new toys for the baby.
- Benefits: New, age-appropriate toys for development.

12. Create a Play Area Near the Baby
- What to Do: Set up a play zone for the toddler near the baby's space.
- Money-Saving Option: Rearrange existing toys and furniture to create the area.
- Benefits: No extra spending, encourages sibling bonding.
- No-Budget Option: Buy new play furniture and baby-safe play mats.
- Benefits: Designated, safe areas for both kids to enjoy.

13. Stock Up on Multipurpose Baby Supplies
- What to Do: Get supplies that work for both children.
- Money-Saving Option: Buy in bulk and use gentle, multipurpose products.
- Benefits: Cuts down on cost and storage space.
- No-Budget Option: Buy specialized products for each child.
- Benefits: Tailored solutions for each child's unique needs.

4. Install Extra Storage for Baby Gear
- What to Do: Add storage solutions for baby items.
- Money-Saving Option: Use baskets, shelves, or storage bins you already have.
- Benefits: Organizes space without spending extra.
- No-Budget Option: Install custom shelving or cabinets.
- Benefits: Sleek, personalized storage for maximum efficiency.

15. Create a Safe Baby Zone for Crawling and Play
- What to Do: Babyproof a safe area for the baby.
- Money-Saving Option: Use items you already have like diy old cribs into baby gates, pillows and blankets, for a soft, safe zone.
- Benefits: Zero cost, creates a safe environment.
- No-Budget Option: Purchase baby playpens and gates.
- Benefits: Fully baby proofed space for peace of mind.

16. Set Up a Family Calendar
- What to Do: Create a calendar to organize family activities and appointments.
- Money-Saving Option: Use a paper calendar or a free app.
- Benefits: Easily tracks schedules without spending extra.
- No-Budget Option: Invest in a large wall-mounted or smart calendar system.
- Benefits: High-tech organization, keeps everyone on the same page.

17. Designate Special Baby-Free Zones for Toddler Time
- What to Do: Create areas where your toddler can have one-on-one attention.
- Money-Saving Option: Rearrange the furniture to set up dedicated toddler areas.
- Benefits: Fosters toddler independence without extra costs.
- No-Budget Option: Create a fully furnished toddler-only playroom.
- Benefits: High-quality play space that gives your toddler special attention.

18. Plan for Minimalist Décor
- What to Do: Keep baby décor simple and functional.
- Money-Saving Option: Use minimal decorations or DIY décor.
- Benefits: Saves money and reduces clutter.
- No-Budget Option: Purchase designer baby décor.
- Benefits: Stylish, personalized nursery with high-quality pieces.

19. Set Up a Toy Rotation System
- What to Do: Rotate toddler's toys to keep them interested.
- Money-Saving Option: Use storage bins to organize toys for easy rotation.
- Benefits: Keeps toys fresh without needing new ones.
- No-Budget Option: Buy new toys regularly for rotation.
- Benefits: Provides consistent excitement with new, stimulating toys.

20. Gather baby items
- What to Do: Gather baby items by swapping or borrowing.
- Money-Saving Option: Join local buy-nothing groups or use hand-me-downs.
- Benefits: Saves a lot of money while still getting essentials.
- No-Budget Option: Buy all new baby gear and accessories.
- Benefits: Brand-new, up-to-date baby items tailored to your preferences.

This list provides practical solutions for setting up your home for a new baby, whether you're looking to save money or invest in higher-end options.

Preparing for each of my babies was more than just getting ready; it became a way to focus on the excitement of meeting my little one. Getting the baby gear set up was a project that kept me motivated and gave me a sense of purpose. As I organized and set up each item, it felt like I was creating a special space for the new chapter of our family.

My pregnancies were never easy, filled with moments that tested me physically and emotionally, but planning for my little one gave me something to look forward to. It was a way to focus on the joy and excitement of meeting my baby, even on the hardest days.

As I prepared, I quickly realized that baby things take up a lot of room, and with limited space, I needed to get organized. I sorted through storage, pulling out items I had saved—those special things with big memories attached. I couldn't keep everything, though; it just wasn't practical. But each time I held something from the past, like a tiny onesie or a well-loved blanket, it brought back memories and reminded me of how far I had come.

I turned to social media to find gently used items, knowing that babies grow so quickly, and most things were barely touched. I was amazed by what I found—items that were nearly new or in perfect condition. When it came to things related to safety or sanitation, I made sure to get those brand new. Insurance helped with some of the essentials, and during tough times, I reached out for assistance through local organizations and, of course, the grandparents. There were moments when it felt hard to ask for help, but I reminded myself that doing my best for my baby was what mattered most. And I believe that when you're trying your best, there's no shame in asking for help. I also made a promise to myself that when I was in a better place, I would give back as much as I could. I've been blessed with so many generous gifts and opportunities, and I believe it's because I've tried to give whenever I can. Whether passing on baby gear, sharing resources, or just offering support, I've seen how we're all in this together. It's a cycle of giving and receiving, and when we lift each other up, it makes the journey a little easier for us all. Preparing for my babies not only helped me get through my pregnancies but also taught me the beauty of community, generosity, and leaning on each other when we need it most.

Chapter 2
Heading to the Hospital

What to Pack for Delivery Day

Packing for the hospital helps ease your mind and promotes quicker healing by ensuring you have personal comforts. While essentials like clothes and toiletries are useful, don't worry if you forget something—the hospital provides everything necessary, just not the personalized items you might want.

1. Witch Hazel + Warm Water for Peri Bottle
-Why: To soothe and heal your perineal area after birth.
-Benefits: Witch hazel reduces pain and swelling, helping with recovery.

2. Hand Pump for Milk
-Why: To stimulate milk production and collect colostrum.
-Benefits: Hand pumps often help you get more colostrum and milk than a regular pump or breastfeeding.

3. Heat Packs (Multiple)
-Why: To relieve pain in various areas.
-Benefits: Helps with sore breasts, clogged ducts, back pain, and cramps.

4. Headphones
-Why: To stay entertained and connected.
-Benefits: Listen to music, movies or podcasts.

5. Extra Long Phone Charger
-Why: Hospital outlets may be far from the bed.
-Benefits: Ensures your devices stay charged without needing to get up.

6. Toiletries (Toothbrush, Deodorant, Q-tips, Face Wipes, Hair Ties)
-Why: To stay fresh.
-Benefits: Keeps you feeling clean and comfortable after labor.

7. Towel and Washcloth
-Why: Hospital towels are often thin and scratchy.
-Benefits: A soft, thick towel provides more comfort for your first postpartum shower.

8. List of Baby Names
-Why: You need to pick out a name before you leave the hospital. -Benefits: Having a list of potential names ready makes the decision process easier when you're tired or overwhelmed.

9. Birth Plan
-Why: To ensure your preferences for labor and delivery are followed.
-Benefits: Clearly communicates your wishes for pain management, interventions, and newborn care.

10. Insurance Card and ID
-Why: For hospital admission and billing.
-Benefits: Ensures a smooth check-in process and prevents billing issues.

11. Baggy, Easy-Fit Dresses
-Why: For comfort post-birth.
-Benefits: Allows easy movement, especially when swollen or sore.

12. Easy-Fit, No-Pressure Period Underwear
-Why: To manage postpartum bleeding comfortably.
-Benefits: Provides better comfort and absorbency than hospital mesh underwear.

13. Nursing Bras
-Why: For comfort while breastfeeding.
-Benefits: Provides easy access for feeding and extra support for your changing breasts.

14. Slippers/ Flip Flops
-Why: Hospital floors can be cold and uncomfortable.
-Benefits: Keeps your feet warm and offers comfort when walking around.

15. Robe
-Why: For easy coverage and warmth.
-Benefits: Ideal for quick cover-ups and comfort during hospital stays.

16. Favorite Snack & Drink
-Why: Hospital options may not suit your taste.
-Benefits: Keeps energy up and provides comfort after delivery.

17. Favorite Blanket & Pillow (Plus Significant Other's Blanket & Pillow)
-Why: Hospital bedding is often uncomfortable for both you and your partner.
-Benefits: Helps you both feel more at home and sleep better.

18. Pictures of Your Other Kids
-Why: For emotional support.
-Benefits: Helps you feel connected to your family during labor.

19. Car Seat with Infant Inserts (Have Base Installed in Car)
-Why: The hospital checks the car seat before your baby can leave.
-Benefits: Infant inserts help your newborn pass the car seat test and provide proper support.

20. Going Home Outfits for Baby, You, & Your Partner
-Why: To ensure everyone is comfortable.
-Benefits: Bring a couple of baby outfits in different sizes, plus comfy clothes for you and your partner.

For three out of four births, I had everything packed and ready—just as planned. The bags were organized, the house was set, and I felt confident that nothing would catch me off guard. I had all the essentials: clothes, diapers, snacks, and even my trusty birth playlist. Still, despite the careful planning, I never quite felt prepared when it was time to head to the hospital. There was always this sense that no matter how much I thought I had covered, something would go awry. And, with my third baby, I found out just how true that was.

The little one had a plan of their own, arriving earlier than expected, without so much as a warning. That was the day we had nothing packed—no bag, no baby clothes, not even a car seat in the car! Of course, I panicked. But in the end, we managed. The hospital had a lot of things ready for us, and they gave me everything from diapers to postpartum supplies. I learned then that sometimes, you just have to ask, and the hospital can provide more than you'd expect.

However, the one thing we hadn't really planned for was a name. We already had one of each—a girl and a boy. So, for our third, we decided to wait until after birth to see if she was a boy or a girl—I was convinced she was a boy because of how my pregnancy was. We were sure we'd just "know" once we saw them. Which was true, but after a week and ten names later. The name we had lined up for a girl, though, was Hazel. It wasn't until we got home that we realized having a Hazen and a Hazel in the same house might've been asking for chaos. The constant mix-up of names started driving us nuts!

To make matters worse, the hospital wouldn't let us get discharged until we filled out the birth certificate paperwork, which included deciding on a name. Talk about pressure! It was less than 24 hours since I'd given birth, and I was still completely out of it. I remember how overwhelming it felt, knowing we had to pick something before we could even leave the hospital.

For a week, we tried what felt like ten different names, trying to see what fit. After endless back-and-forth, we finally settled on Lola, which totally fits her. It's funny how something like that can slip through the cracks when you're in the thick of planning. To this day, I still need to get the name officially changed!

If I could give any advice from that experience, it's this: make sure you have a few names picked out ahead of time, no matter how confident you feel in your choice. And while packing every possible thing is nice, just remember the hospital has plenty on hand—you can always ask for what you need!

Coordinating Childcare for Your Other Children

1. Daily Routine List: Write out each child's daily schedule, from wake-up to bedtime.
   -Benefit: Helps caregivers maintain consistency, making the transition smoother for your children.

2. Meal Preferences List: Include foods your kids like and dislike.
   -Benefit: Ensures they eat well and avoid unnecessary stress during your absence.

3. Frozen Meals & Snacks: Prepare and freeze their favorite meals and stock up on snacks.
   -Benefit: Caregivers have easy, ready-made meals, and kids get the comfort of familiar foods.

4. House Rules List: Clarify places the kids can and can't go and activities that are off-limits.
   -Benefit: Keeps boundaries clear and helps caregivers manage the children safely.

5. Emergency Contact List: Provide numbers for family members, doctors, and close friends.
   -Benefit: Offers quick access to support in case of unforeseen events.

6. Behavioral Guidelines List: Include how you prefer the children be disciplined and comforted.
   -Benefit: Reduces confusion and maintains consistency in parenting approaches.

7. Plan for Emotional Support: Include ways to comfort your children when they feel sad or anxious.
   -Benefit: Helps caregivers know how to emotionally support your children.

8. Backup Child Care Contacts: Arrange for secondary caregivers in case the primary ones are unavailable.
   -Benefit: Provides flexibility and reassurance if plans change unexpectedly.

9. Favorite Toys/Blankets Ready: Ensure favorite items are clean, available, and have fresh batteries if needed.
   -Benefit: Familiar objects can provide comfort during a stressful time.

10. Activities for Overwhelm: Suggest calming activities or safe spaces they can retreat to if things get out of control.
   -Benefit: Gives children an outlet for managing stress and helps caregivers redirect energy.

11. Hair Braiding/Styling: Pre-braid or style their hair so it requires minimal attention.
   -Benefit: Reduces morning stress for both the children and caregivers.

12. Arrange Playdates: Schedule playdates with friends or family members.
   -Benefit: Keeps the children entertained and engaged with familiar faces.

13. School/Daycare Information: Provide the caregivers with details about pickup, drop-off, and special instructions.
   --Benefit: Ensures the school routine isn't disrupted and keeps transitions smooth.

14. Pack for Emergencies: Prepare a bag with clothes, diapers, medications, and other essentials for emergencies.
   -Benefit: Caregivers can handle unexpected situations easily without scrambling for supplies.

15. Bedtime Routine Checklist: List the steps for bedtime, including favorite stories, songs, or bedtime rituals.
   -Benefit: Keeps bedtime familiar and soothing, helping children feel secure in your absence.

16. Medical Information List: Provide a list of allergies, medications, and health conditions.
   -Benefit: Ensures that caregivers are well-informed and can act quickly if necessary.

17. Positive Language Guidelines: Include phrases or approaches you prefer when your kids are being spoken to.
   -Benefit: Ensures that children are treated with the same care and consistency they are used to.

18. Backup Clothing: Set out a week's worth of clothes to avoid any confusion about what they should wear.
   -Benefit: Prevents unnecessary decision-making for caregivers and ensures children are dressed appropriately.

19. Pet Care Instructions: If you have pets, provide a detailed care list for feeding, walks, and other needs.
   -Benefit: Ensures the pet routine continues smoothly, preventing additional chaos.

20.Favorite Shows, Movies, and Video Games: Create a list of approved screen time options, including their favorite shows, movies, and video games.
   -Benefit: Provides caregivers with easy ways to keep the children entertained, while ensuring content is appropriate and familiar to them.

These preparations ensure the children stay comfortable, routines remain consistent, and caregivers have clear guidance, making your hospital stay smoother for everyone involved. Whether it's school, daycare, or family members stepping in, the standards we hold matter more than we often realize. The truth is, if you let things slide and those instructions aren't followed, it won't take long before your words lose weight. Eventually, your children will notice too, and they'll start pushing back, realizing that what you say isn't always backed up.

I learned this lesson early with my children, especially as I had them so close together. I had to trust the people watching my kids, knowing that their approach might differ from mine. But I needed to feel confident that they respected my wishes enough to stick to the plan—even if it wasn't their way of doing things. With each birth, I found myself relying on family and friends more and more, and each time it was a test of that trust.

For my third child, everything seemed to go wrong. That baby came early, and I hadn't even packed a hospital bag. My other children needed care, and in the rush, I didn't have time to get my daughter's hair braided, something I always did to make things easier for everyone. Two days into the chaos, my dad brought the kids to the hospital to see us. From the moment I saw my daughter walking down that hall, her hair wild and untamed, it brought tears to my eyes—not out of frustration, but pure joy.

My dad, clearly feeling defeated, looked at me and said, "I'm so sorry, honey. I tried brushing it." The exhaustion in his voice was clear, but so was his effort. He had tried, really tried. I could see the love and care he had poured into looking after my children, even if things weren't exactly how I would've done them. That moment was bitter and sweet all at once. It reminded me that while things might not always go perfectly, the people I trusted had done their best to keep my kids safe and happy.

In the end, that's what matters most. Parenting isn't about perfection. It's about setting boundaries, following through, and finding those who will love and respect you enough to honor the way you choose to raise your children—even if things don't always go according to plan.

Handling Multiple Births in a Short Time Frame

1. Establish a Routine Early: Set up a daily schedule for feeding, naps, and playtime.
   -Benefit: Creates structure, helping you manage your time and reducing stress for both parents and babies.

2. Prepare Meals in Advance: Stockpile frozen meals and snacks ahead of time.
   -Benefit: Saves time during busy days and ensures you can easily feed the whole family without extra effort.

3. Delegate Tasks: Ask for help from family, friends, or a babysitter.
   -Benefit: Lightens your workload, allowing you to focus on bonding with your babies and avoiding burnout.

4. Invest in Double (or Triple) Baby Gear: Buy essentials like double strollers, car seats, and cribs for each baby.
   -Benefit: Ensures each baby has what they need and simplifies outings and transportation.

5. Sync Naps: Encourage your babies to nap at the same time.
   -Benefit: Gives you a block of downtime to rest, clean, or attend to other tasks.

6. Breastfeed Simultaneously: If breastfeeding, nurse both babies at once using a twin nursing pillow.
   -Benefit: Saves time and can help establish a shared feeding routine.

7. Create a Feeding Station: Set up a space with bottles, formula, pump, and burp cloths.
   -Benefit: Keeps everything organized and accessible, making feeding easier, especially during late nights.

8. Accept Help When Offered: Don't hesitate to accept help from others, especially for chores.
   -Benefit: Frees up your time and energy, allowing you to focus on your children and yourself.

9. Meal Train: Ask friends or family to organize a meal train after each birth.
   -Benefit: Ensures you have home-cooked meals during the early postpartum weeks when you're juggling newborn care.

10. Organize a Play Area for Toddlers: Have a safe space with toys and activities for older kids to entertain themselves.
   -Benefit: Keeps older children engaged and allows you to focus on the babies when needed.

11. Establish Quiet Time: Introduce a quiet time during the day where toddlers can relax or nap.
   -Benefit: Provides you with some calm and a break from constant noise and activity.

12.Prioritize Sleep: Take naps when your babies sleep, and consider sleep training methods when they're ready.
   -Benefit: Helps you recover from sleep deprivation, boosting your energy and mood.

13. Rotate Caregiving Duties: Alternate nighttime feedings or diaper changes with your partner.
   -Benefit: Prevents one parent from becoming overwhelmed and ensures both parents get some rest.

14. Babywearing: Use slings or baby carriers to wear one or both babies while managing household tasks.
   -Benefit: Keeps your hands free and babies close, fostering bonding and making multitasking easier.

15. Keep Diaper Stations Stocked: Set up changing stations in different rooms with all essentials—diapers, wipes, and creams.

   -Benefit: Saves time and reduces the hassle of searching for supplies during diaper changes.

16. Designate "Baby-Free" Time: Schedule time for self-care or a date night with your partner.

   -Benefit: Allows you to recharge and strengthens your relationship with your partner amidst the chaos.

17. Group Doctor Visits: Schedule pediatric appointments for both babies at the same time.

   Benefit: Saves time and reduces the number of trips to the doctor.

18. Batch Baby Laundry: Wash all baby clothes, bibs, and blankets together in larger loads.

   -Benefit: Streamlines laundry tasks, cutting down on time spent sorting and washing.

19. Join a Support Group for Multiples: Connect with other parents who have multiples for advice and camaraderie.

   -Benefit: Provides emotional support, shared tips, and a sense of community with those who understand your situation.

20. Stay Organized with Lists: Keep a running list of baby supplies, appointments, and feeding times.

   -Benefit: Helps you stay on top of your responsibilities and reduces the chances of forgetting important tasks.

Handling multiple births close together can feel overwhelming, but these strategies provide structure, reduce stress, and make managing your household and children much more feasible.

When my first daughter was born, she never wanted to be away from me. For the first few months, she was constantly in a front pack, snug against my chest, whether I was cooking, cleaning, or just trying to steal a moment of rest. It became second nature to move through my day with her right there. I didn't mind it at all—it was our time to bond, and she was happiest when she was close. It's funny how those moments made me feel needed, but also, in a way, grounded.

As much as I loved having her near, I quickly realized that I thrive on having a routine, especially a solid sleep schedule. When I was pregnant with my other children, I would use nap time to catch a short break myself, recharging to make it through the day. But now, with more kids and no pregnancy naps, I use that precious time to get things done and prepare for what's coming next. Nap time has become the cornerstone of my day, where I can reset, clean up, and organize the chaos so when the kids wake, things run smoothly.

But when we get off schedule, everything feels like chaos. It's amazing how quickly things can spiral. One missed nap or an off day, and suddenly it feels like we're running in circles, everyone is cranky, and nothing gets done. That's why I like to rotate our routines and change things up just enough to keep the kids engaged and excited. Whether it's switching up activities or moving lunch outdoors, a little variety keeps everyone from getting bored. Still, the core of our days always goes back to that structure, because without it, the house falls apart.

If I don't prepare the night before, I feel the stress start to build the moment we wake up. The kids sense it too. Suddenly, we're running late, and everything feels harder than it needs to be. But when I've taken the time to set things up ahead of time—laying out clothes, prepping breakfast, stocking the diaper station—the day usually flows smoothly. The kids are happier, more helpful, and I feel like I'm in control. Those mornings when everything is ready and we're on time, it's like a victory, no matter what the rest of the day brings.

But emotions can shift fast with kids, especially in those small moments that throw you off. Like when you go to change a blowout diaper and toss it in the trash, only to reach for the wipes and realize you're out. It's a moment of pure panic and frustration, like the universe is playing a cruel joke on you. But that's when I remind myself—it's all about setting up your future self for success. When I take a few extra minutes the night before to restock and prepare, I'm making sure tomorrow's me can handle whatever comes. And when I do, it makes me feel pretty good, like I'm taking care of myself just as much as my kids.

It's not always perfect, and chaos is always lurking just around the corner, but when things are in place, everything seems to click. The kids are content, and I'm able to take a breath, knowing that we're all on track. It's those moments when I feel like I've got this. Even if the blowouts and messes come, at least I'm ready for them.

Chapter 3
Being in the Hospital

Navigating Labor and Delivery

1. Call the Hospital in Advance: Give the labor and delivery unit a heads-up before arriving.
   -Benefit: Ensures they're prepared for your arrival, potentially reducing wait times and easing the check-in process.

2. Bring a Gift for the Staff (around 15 people): Consider bringing a small token like trinkets, treats, or thank-you notes for the team.
   -Benefit: Shows appreciation, and a happy, appreciated staff tends to offer more personalized and attentive care.

3. Research Hospital Policies: Look up the hospital's policies on birth plans, visitors, and pain management.
   -Benefit: Helps you feel prepared and reduces surprises during the delivery process, allowing for a smoother experience.

4. Discuss Pain Management Options in Advance: Understand your options for pain relief (epidural, natural birth, etc.) and make a plan.
   -Benefit: Reduces anxiety and helps you stay in control of your labor preferences.

5. Tour the Hospital: Take a hospital tour, either virtually or in person, to familiarize yourself with the layout.
   -Benefit: Eases nerves by making you more comfortable with your surroundings on the big day.

6. Stay Flexible: Be ready to adjust to the unexpected during labor, as things don't always go as planned.

   -Benefit: Lowers stress and helps you feel more in control when plans change during delivery.

7. Create a Flexible Birth Plan: Draft a birth plan, but be prepared for it to change if necessary.

   -Benefit: Clarifies your preferences while maintaining flexibility for unexpected changes.

8. Talk to Other Moms: Chat with friends or join a mom's group to hear their experiences and advice.

   -Benefit: Offers emotional support and practical tips from those who have been through labor and delivery.

9. Take Prenatal Classes: Enroll in a childbirth class to learn breathing techniques, positions, and what to expect.

   -Benefit: Builds confidence in handling contractions and gives you tools to manage labor effectively.

10. Prepare Mentally for Hospital Staff: Understand that some nurses and staff may not have children themselves, so they might not fully understand what certain things feel like.

   -Benefit: Encourages patience and understanding, making the experience smoother for everyone involved.

11. Hydrate Leading Up to Labor: Drink plenty of water in the days leading up to your due date.

   -Benefit: Staying hydrated can make labor easier and reduce the chance of complications.

12. Keep Your Doctor Informed: Make sure your OB-GYN or midwife knows your birth plan and any concerns.

   -Benefit: Ensures they are aligned with your wishes and can support you during delivery.

13. Use Visualization Techniques: Practice visualization or meditation to stay calm and focused.
   -Benefit: Helps manage anxiety and creates a more relaxed mindset going into labor.

14. Bring Items for Comfort: Pack personal items like a pillow, favorite blanket, or essential oils.
   -Benefit: Makes the hospital feel more like home, increasing comfort during labor.

15. Delegate Responsibilities: Assign tasks to your partner or support person, like handling communication with family or managing paperwork.
   -Benefit: Reduces the mental load and allows you to focus on the delivery.

16. Enjoy Being Pampered: Let the hospital staff take care of you, from meals to monitoring your vitals.
   -Benefit: Allows you to rest and recuperate, enjoying the attention and care.

17. Take Walks if Possible: If allowed, walk around during early labor to help speed up the process.
   -Benefit: Encourages labor progression and can help manage pain naturally.

18. Bring Snacks for After Delivery: Hospital food may not always hit the spot, so pack your favorite snacks.
   -Benefit: Keeps your energy levels up, especially after the hard work of labor.

19. Limit Visitors as Needed: Decide in advance who can visit during and after delivery.
   -Benefit: Provides a calm, restful environment for you to bond with your baby.

20. Celebrate Small Wins: During labor, celebrate milestones like dilation progress or baby positioning.

   -Benefit: Boosts morale and helps you feel in control and proud of your journey.

With each birth, I learned a little more about what to expect, even though none of my doctors ever made it in time. My first delivery set the tone for the rest. The doctor missed it by just a minute, bursting into the room out of breath, having sprinted down the hallway as fast as he could. He was panting, apologizing, but by then, my baby had already arrived. It was such a chaotic, surreal moment, but in the end, it didn't really matter. There were still nurses and other doctors surrounding me, making sure everything went smoothly. It was like stepping into another world—a place where time slowed down, where I was both there and not there, riding the waves of contractions and trying to focus on the moment.

Every time, I thought I knew what to expect, but labor has a way of throwing curveballs. There were moments when I would get these false assurances, like someone would tell me something about what was coming next, and it wouldn't quite line up with reality. My husband, thankfully, kept me grounded. "They've never been through this themselves," he'd remind me when I'd start to get worked up over a comment or an instruction that didn't feel right. He was right. A lot of the time, it was staff who hadn't experienced childbirth firsthand, and their advice didn't always match what I was feeling in my body.

With each birth, I gathered new lessons. After my third baby, I learned a critical one about pain management. Half of my epidural didn't work, and it was unbearable. I was in so much pain, barely hanging on. I remember them checking my numbness with ice, asking if I could feel it, and that's when they figured out that the medicine hadn't taken on one side of my body. They turned me, using gravity to get the medication to the right place, but it took so long, and I was already deep in labor. So, for my fourth birth, I wasn't taking any chances. The moment the epidural was administered, I asked for ice and made sure I was numb on both sides. I wasn't going to wait until I was in agony again to check.

By that fourth birth, my husband had become an expert at following my contractions on the monitor. He'd stand by my side, calmly watching the lines rise and fall, telling me when a contraction was coming and when it was starting to ease off. It was comforting, having someone next to me who understood the process as well as I did by then. Even though my doctor missed that delivery too, I felt more in control. My husband and I had figured out our own rhythm by then, and between the two of us and the incredible nurses, we managed just fine.

Each experience was different, but in the end, I always felt supported. My doctor may have missed all my births, but I never felt alone. The team around me knew what they were doing, and with each new delivery, I grew more confident in trusting myself and the process. What mattered most was that I left the hospital each time with a healthy baby in my arms, and that's something I'll always be grateful for.

Hospital Recovery Tips for the Busy Mom

1. Use Witch Hazel in the Peri Bottle: Add a little alcohol-free witch hazel to your peri bottle for soothing relief during postpartum care.
   -Benefit: Helps reduce swelling and speeds up healing, providing comfort during recovery.

2. Ask for Extra Supplies: Don't hesitate to ask the nurses for additional mesh underwear, pads, or ice packs before you leave.
   -Benefit: Ensures you have enough supplies to stay comfortable at home without needing to go shopping right away.

3. Accept Help Even If You Don't Think You Need It: When family or friends offer assistance, accept it graciously, even if you feel you can manage.
   -Benefit: Allows you to rest and recover more effectively, avoiding burnout and exhaustion.

4. Don't Be Embarrassed by Postpartum Realities: Childbirth is messy, but it's natural. Don't feel embarrassed by the "grossness" of recovery.
   -Benefit: Helps you feel more at ease, making it easier to communicate your needs to medical staff and family.

5. Limit Visitors If Needed: Don't be afraid to say no to friends and family who want to visit if you're not feeling up to it.
   -Benefit: Provides you with the peace and quiet needed to rest and bond with your newborn.

6. Rest as Much as Possible: Take advantage of any quiet moments in the hospital to rest or nap.
   -Benefit: Aids in faster healing and prepares you for the sleepless nights ahead.

7. Stay Hydrated: Drink plenty of water and fluids to stay hydrated, especially if you're breastfeeding.
   -Benefit: Helps your body recover and supports milk production.

8. Take Short Walks When Allowed: If your doctor permits, take short walks around the hospital to promote circulation.
   -Benefit: Helps prevent blood clots and can reduce soreness.

9. Use a Postpartum Belly Wrap: Consider using a postpartum belly wrap for support and comfort.
   -Benefit: Offers abdominal support, reduces swelling, and can help you feel more secure when moving around.

10. Communicate Your Pain Levels: Don't try to tough it out. Let the nurses know if you're in pain or uncomfortable.
   -Benefit: Ensures you receive adequate pain relief, making recovery smoother.

11. Set Up a Feeding Station: Have a dedicated spot with all your breastfeeding or bottle-feeding supplies within reach.
   -Benefit: Saves time and effort, making feedings more efficient and comfortable.

12. Bring Comfortable Clothes: Pack loose, soft clothing for your hospital stay, like a robe or pajamas.
   -Benefit: Provides comfort and easy access for nursing or skin-to-skin contact.

13. Use the Hospital Lactation Consultant: Take advantage of the hospital's lactation consultant for breastfeeding tips and support.
   -Benefit: Helps you establish a good breastfeeding routine and addresses any initial concerns.

14. Focus on One Day at a Time: Recovery is a process. Don't overwhelm yourself by thinking too far ahead.
   -Benefit: Reduces stress and anxiety, allowing you to focus on immediate recovery needs.

15. Bring Your Favorite Snacks: Hospital food may not always meet your preferences. Pack some of your favorite snacks.
   -Benefit: Keeps your energy up and helps you feel more at home.

16. Prioritize Skin-to-Skin Time: Spend as much time as possible holding your baby skin-to-skin.
   -Benefit: Promotes bonding, helps regulate your baby's temperature, and supports breastfeeding.

17. Practice Deep Breathing or Meditation: Use deep breathing exercises or meditation to stay calm and relaxed.
   -Benefit: Helps manage stress and can speed up recovery by promoting relaxation.

18. Plan for Nighttime Support: Arrange for someone to stay with you overnight if allowed, whether it's a partner, friend, or family member.
   -Benefit: Provides extra help and emotional support during challenging nighttime hours.

19. Don't Feel Rushed to Leave: If you're not feeling ready, don't feel pressured to leave the hospital.
   -Benefit: Gives you time to feel more stable and confident in your recovery before heading home.

20. Prepare for Emotional Ups and Downs: Understand that hormonal changes can lead to mood swings or baby blues.
   -Benefit: Helps you recognize these feelings as normal, making it easier to ask for support if needed.

All of my babies were born during the COVID-19 pandemic, a time that made things even more complicated. We had to be incredibly strict about who could visit and see them. So many people didn't understand why we were being cautious, and some even made us feel terrible for enforcing boundaries. But I'm so glad we stood our ground. Keeping our babies safe was our top priority, and I have no regrets about being selective about visitors. It was hard to deal with the judgment, but looking back, we did what was best for our family.

Even before the pandemic, we had strong feelings about how we wanted things to go, especially with our first baby. I remember the raised eyebrows and the quiet comments when we decided that we only wanted my husband and me in the delivery room. People thought we were being selfish, but it turned out to be one of the best decisions we ever made. It was magical. Just the two of us, together, bringing our first child into the world. There was a calmness to it, and it allowed us to share that moment without distractions. I wouldn't change a thing.

After my second child, though, I learned some hard lessons about accepting help. I wanted to take a shower, and in my mind, I thought I was fine. I felt strong enough and turned down help from the nurses. But as soon as I stood up, I felt off-balance, and then I fell. Right before I could get into the shower, I hit the ground, and shortly after, I started throwing up. It was a huge wake-up call. I had pushed myself too soon, thinking I could handle it all, but I was wrong. I wish I had taken it easy and accepted the help that was being offered. Sometimes, being strong means knowing when to rest.

One thing I've always cherished is skin-to-skin contact. It really is magical, and the science behind it backs it up. Holding my baby against my chest wasn't just about bonding; it helped regulate their body temperature, heart rate, and breathing. It even supported breastfeeding and helped us both stay calm. It's amazing how something so simple can have such profound benefits.

But not everything was perfect after my second child. I decided to get the Depo shot as birth control, and it ended up throwing me into postpartum depression. I could feel myself disconnecting from my baby. I wanted so badly to bond, to feel that love and connection, but something was off. I couldn't explain it to anyone, but inside, it felt like I had this burning ball of emotion, ready to explode at any moment, and I couldn't break free of it. My moods were extreme, and no matter how hard I tried, I just couldn't get out of that dark space. I remember feeling helpless, desperate to connect but unable to.

When the effects of the shot finally wore off, I felt like a heavy blanket had been lifted off me. I could breathe again, feel again. But it didn't happen overnight. It took a lot of work—meditation, self-realization, and some serious self-care. I had to dig deep to heal and find myself again. Looking back, I realize how much that experience taught me about mental health and the importance of being gentle with myself.

Through it all, I've learned that trusting myself and setting boundaries is crucial, whether it's keeping my babies safe during a pandemic or knowing when to ask for help. Parenting isn't always easy, and sometimes the hardest lessons are the ones that make you stronger in the end.

Introducing the New Baby to Their Siblings

1. Encourage Siblings to Talk to the Baby in the Belly
   Have siblings talk or sing to your belly daily. You can also use a stethoscope or a tube to amplify their voices.
   -Benefit: Babies can hear sounds from around 18 weeks gestation. Hearing their sibling's voice helps them recognize and bond with them after birth, making the transition smoother.

2. Teach About Calm, Soft Hands
   Practice using "soft hands" on a doll or stuffed animal, showing them how to gently touch and pat. Reinforce the behavior by praising them when they use gentle touches.
   -Benefit: Prepares older siblings to use gentle touches, preventing accidental harm and teaching them to interact lovingly, fostering positive sibling relationships.

3. Explain Where They Can and Cannot Touch the Baby
   Show your older child where it's safe to touch the baby, like their feet or back, and explain why the face or head should be avoided. Use role-playing to reinforce this.
   -Benefit: Clear boundaries reduce anxiety for both siblings and parents. Knowing safe spots to touch helps siblings feel more confident in interacting safely.

4. Use Positive Language About Being a Big Sibling
   Use phrases like "You're such a great big sibling" and "The baby loves you so much." Celebrate their new role and give them small responsibilities.
   -Benefit: Builds self-esteem and gives them a sense of pride and responsibility, reducing jealousy and negative behavior.

5. Create a 'Big Sibling' Kit
Put together a small gift bag with items like books, a special "big sibling" shirt, or toys they enjoy. Present it to them when they meet the baby for the first time.
-Benefit: Helps older siblings feel celebrated and included in the baby's arrival, making them feel special and valued.

6. Read Books About New Siblings Together
Choose books about becoming a big sibling and read them together, discussing the story afterward to see how they feel about their own upcoming role.
-Benefit: Stories help children understand and normalize their feelings about the new baby, providing language and context for this big change.

7. Discuss Family and Togetherness
Talk about how the new baby is part of your family and emphasize that everyone plays an important role. Use phrases like, "We're a team" or "We take care of each other."
-Benefit: Reduces feelings of exclusion and reinforces that the baby's arrival is a positive change for everyone.

8. Involve Siblings in Baby Preparations
Allow them to help set up the nursery, choose baby clothes, or decorate the room. This gives them a sense of ownership and involvement.
-Benefit: Makes them feel included in the process, reducing jealousy and fostering positive feelings toward the new baby.

9. Talk About the Baby's Needs and Why They Cry
Explain in simple terms why babies cry, like hunger or needing a diaper change. Reassure them that the baby isn't upset with them.
-Benefit: Helps siblings understand and respond calmly to crying, reducing anxiety and promoting empathy.

10. Plan Special One-on-One Time

Schedule time alone with each child, even if it's just a short activity like reading a book or playing their favorite game.

-Benefit: Reassures them that they are still important and loved, reducing rivalry and feelings of neglect.

11. Encourage Siblings to Sing or Read to the Baby

Teach them simple lullabies or have them read a short story to the baby. Make it part of the bedtime routine if possible.

-Benefit: Promotes bonding and language development for the baby while boosting the older sibling's confidence and connection.

12. Create a Safe Space for Sibling Emotions

Set aside a specific time each day to talk about how they're feeling. Use emotion cards or a feelings chart to help them express themselves.

-Benefit: Acknowledging and validating their feelings fosters emotional security and helps them process complex emotions healthily.

13. Include Siblings in Baby Care (With Supervision)

Let them hand you diapers, choose the baby's outfit, or help with bath time under close supervision.

-Benefit: Makes them feel helpful and involved, promoting positive sibling interaction and reducing feelings of exclusion.

14. Model Calm and Gentle Interactions

Demonstrate calm, gentle behaviors when holding or caring for the baby, using a soothing voice and slow movements. Encourage siblings to mimic these actions.

-Benefit: Sets a powerful example for siblings to follow, promoting calm and loving interactions with the baby.

15. Avoid Comparing Siblings to the Baby

Focus on each child's strengths and unique qualities instead of making comparisons. Use statements like, "You're amazing at drawing," rather than "The baby needs a lot of attention right now."

-Benefit: Helps maintain each child's unique identity and self-esteem, preventing feelings of competition and jealousy.

16. Allow Siblings to Express Discomfort or Frustration

Let them know it's okay to feel upset or frustrated. Use phrases like, "It's okay to feel mad that the baby is crying a lot. It's hard for everyone right now."

-Benefit: Encouraging open communication helps children feel heard and understood, reducing negative behavior and emotional outbursts.

17. Set Up a Sibling Celebration

Plan a small party or special meal to celebrate the big sibling role, involving them in choosing decorations or planning a family activity.

-Benefit: Makes them feel important and cherished, reinforcing positive associations with the new baby.

18. Show Old Photos of When They Were a Baby

Look through old baby photos and videos together. Share stories about when they were little and how excited you were to have them.

-Benefit: Helps them relate to the newborn, fostering empathy and understanding of the baby's needs.

19. Use Baby Dolls for Role-Playing

Use a baby doll to demonstrate how to hold and care for a baby. Let siblings practice with the doll and ask questions about the baby's needs.

-Benefit: Allows siblings to practice gentle behaviors and express any concerns or fears they might have about the new baby.

20. Discuss How Babies Know and Recognize Family Members
   Explain that the baby will know and love them because of their voice and presence. Encourage them to speak softly and spend time around the baby.
   -Benefit: Strengthens the sibling bond and makes the older child feel valued and important in the baby's life.

When we found out we were expecting our first baby together, my stepson, Skylar, had been an only child in both households for five years. We knew this was going to be a big adjustment for him, so we made a point of including him in the pregnancy as much as possible. We got him "Big Brother" shirts, talked about what it meant to have a new sibling, and shared how important his role would be. Even though he didn't quite have a sense of time, as my due date got closer, we noticed he became more clingy, wanting extra cuddles and attention.

Skylar would talk, sing, read books, and even tell jokes to my belly. We practiced soft hands and gentle touches with his Lilly bear, getting him used to the idea of being around a tiny, fragile baby. When my daughter, Lilly, was finally born, we were excited and nervous for their first meeting.

The day after she was born, Skylar came to the hospital to meet his baby sister. He walked into the room with a big smile on his face, wearing his "Big Brother" shirt. We sat together on the hospital bed, and I carefully placed Lilly in his arms. Skylar looked down at her, his eyes wide with wonder. With his practiced soft hands, he gently held her tiny body and said, "Hi, Lilly, I'm your big brother, Skylar." At that moment, Lilly, just a day old, smiled for the first time.

It was like she knew who he was, recognizing his voice from all the months he had spent talking and singing to her. That smile was magical, and from that day on, their bond was incredible. They've been inseparable when he is with us ever since. Skylar took on his big brother role with pride, always wanting to help and be near his sister.

Introducing my younger children to their siblings, however, was a different story. They didn't quite understand the concept of a new baby in the same way Skylar did. At first, they were curious and calm, but it didn't take long for them to test boundaries. They would sometimes try to hit or sit on the baby or even offer snacks that definitely weren't safe for an infant. Those early interactions always had to be supervised closely.

I started to notice how they could be together for longer and longer each time without issues, learning to be gentle and loving just like we had practiced. Despite the rough beginnings, those bonds have grown just as deep. Watching them interact now, you'd never guess there was ever a moment of struggle.

It's in those early days and moments that memories are made, not just for the baby, but for the older siblings as well. They may not remember every detail, but they will always feel the love, the connection, and the special role they played in welcoming a new family member. And sometimes, that's all that really matters.

Chapter 4
Surviving the Newborn Stage

Adjusting to Life with a Newborn

1. Establish a Nighttime Routine Early
   Implement a simple bedtime routine, like a bath, feeding, and lullaby.
   -Benefit: Helps the baby distinguish between day and night, leading to better sleep patterns over time.

2. Utilize Swaddling
   Swaddle the baby snugly to recreate the womb-like environment.
   -Benefit: Reduces the startle reflex, helping the baby sleep longer and more peacefully.

3. Accept Help from Family and Friends
   Allow others to cook meals, clean, or babysit older kids.
   -Benefit: Frees up time for you to rest and bond with the baby, reducing stress and exhaustion.

4. Practice Skin-to-Skin Contact
   Spend time holding the baby skin-to-skin.
   -Benefit: Promotes bonding, regulates the baby's body temperature, and helps establish breastfeeding.

5. Use a White Noise Machine
   Play white noise during naps and nighttime.
   - Benefit: Mimics the sounds of the womb, soothing the baby and encouraging deeper sleep.

6. Set Up a Feeding Station
   Create a dedicated spot with water, snacks, burp cloths, and a book or phone for entertainment.
   -Benefit: Keeps everything you need close by, making feedings more comfortable and less stressful.

7. Incorporate Tummy Time Daily
   Place the baby on their tummy for a few minutes each day.
   - Benefit: Strengthens neck and shoulder muscles, promoting motor development and preventing flat spots.

8. Follow Baby's Cues
   Learn to recognize the baby's hunger, tiredness, and discomfort cues.
   -Benefit: Helps you respond promptly to the baby's needs, fostering a secure attachment.

9. Take Short Walks Outside
   Go for short walks with the baby in a stroller or carrier.
   -Benefit: Exposure to fresh air and sunlight improves mood and can help both of you reset during fussy periods.

10. Use a Baby Carrier
   Wear the baby in a front pack during the day.
   -Benefit: Allows you to be hands-free while keeping the baby close, fostering bonding and soothing the baby.

11. Join a New Parent Group
   Connect with other parents of newborns in person or online.
   -Benefit: Provides emotional support, sharing of advice, and a sense of community.

12. Create a Calm Environment
   Keep lights dim and noise low during nighttime feedings.
   -Benefit: Helps the baby stay calm and go back to sleep more easily after waking.

13. Prioritize Self-Care
   Take short breaks to shower, eat, or nap when the baby is sleeping.
   -Benefit: Prevents burnout and helps you feel more refreshed and capable.

14. Use a Nursing Pillow
   Use a pillow to support the baby during breastfeeding or bottle-feeding.
   -Benefit: Reduces strain on your arms and back, making feeding sessions more comfortable.

15. Track Baby's Feeding and Sleep Patterns
   Use an app or notebook to record feedings, diapers, and sleep.
   -Benefit: Helps you identify patterns and ensures the baby is feeding and sleeping enough.

16. Have a Flexible Mindset
   Be prepared to adapt plans and routines as needed.
   -Benefit: Reduces frustration and helps you respond to the baby's changing needs.

17. Stock Up on Essentials
   Keep plenty of diapers, wipes, and snacks for yourself.
   -Benefit: Avoids last-minute trips to the store, reducing stress.

18. Keep a Postpartum Care Kit Handy
   Include items like pain relief, ice packs, and peri bottles.
   -Benefit: Promotes your physical recovery, allowing you to care for the baby more comfortably.

19. Limit Visitors Initially
   Keep visits short and to a minimum.
   -Benefit: Allows you to bond with the baby without feeling overwhelmed or pressured to host.

20. Sing to the Baby
  Sing lullabies or talk to the baby in a soothing voice.
  -Benefit: Helps calm the baby, stimulates brain development, and strengthens your bond.

With each baby, the newborn stage got a little easier, but it was never without its challenges. I remember with my first, feeling like I was constantly worried about everything—if she was breathing, if I was doing things right, or if I could even figure out what she needed. I'd watch her tiny chest rise and fall and smell her head, and in those moments, I'd feel a sense of calm. It was as if the weight of those worries lifted, even if just for a second, and I knew that as long as I was doing my best with unconditional love, we would be okay.

Each time I'd get overwhelmed, I'd think of that song, "It Won't Be Like This for Long," and hum it in my head, reminding myself that these sleepless nights and endless diaper changes wouldn't last forever. It seemed like forever at the time, but looking back, it really was just a short season. Whenever I wasn't sure what to do, I'd reach out—whether it was reading books, searching online, or calling the doctor. And every time, I found an answer, a new way to soothe, or just reassurance that I was doing fine.

By the time my second, third and forth babies came, I had a little more confidence. I'd learned what worked for us and knew the rhythms of those early days. But even then, there were still moments of doubt and exhaustion. I'd look at them, smell their sweet baby scent, and remember that these challenges were temporary. The days were long but the years so short, and every time I'd hold them close, I knew it would all be worth it.

Managing the Needs of Different-Aged Kids

1. Create Individual Routines for Each Child
   Tailor routines for each child's age and needs.
   -Benefit: Provides structure and security, helping children thrive with predictable patterns.

2. Implement a Family Calendar
   Use a visual family calendar for activities and appointments.
   -Benefit: Keeps everyone on the same page and prevents scheduling conflicts.

3. Prioritize One-on-One Time
   Spend focused time with each child, even if brief.
   -Benefit: Strengthens individual relationships and helps each child feel valued.

4. Encourage Sibling Bonding Activities
   Plan activities like board games or storytime that they can do together.
   -Benefit: Fosters a sense of teamwork and helps siblings build a strong bond.

5. Use Visual Schedules for Younger Kids
   Display daily activities and routines using pictures.
   -Benefit: Helps young children understand the day's flow and reduces anxiety.

6. Create a Designated Quiet Time
   Establish a daily period for quiet activities like reading or puzzles.
   -Benefit: Promotes self-regulation and provides a break for everyone.

7. Set Up Independent Play Areas
   Have separate play areas for each age group.
   -Benefit: Keeps kids engaged with age-appropriate activities and reduces conflicts.

8. Involve Older Kids in Caregiving
   Assign simple tasks, like fetching a diaper or singing to the baby.
   -Benefit: Builds responsibility and makes them feel included in family care.

9. Implement Positive Reinforcement
   Reward good behavior with praise or small incentives.
   -Benefit: Encourages positive behavior and reinforces good habits.

10. Rotate Toys and Activities
   Swap out toys and activities every few weeks.
   -Benefit: Keeps kids interested and engaged, preventing boredom.

11. Teach Conflict Resolution Skills
   Role-play scenarios where kids can practice resolving conflicts.
   -Benefit: Helps children learn to handle disagreements peacefully and independently.

12. Use a Baby Monitor for Safety
   Keep a baby monitor in common areas while attending to older kids.
   -Benefit: Allows you to monitor the baby while managing the needs of the older children.

13. Plan Age-Appropriate Outings
   Choose activities that cater to each child's interests, like parks or museums.
   -Benefit: Makes outings enjoyable for everyone and supports learning and exploration.

14. Establish a Family Meal Routine
   Plan regular family meals where everyone sits together.
   -Benefit: Promotes family bonding and teaches healthy eating habits.

15. Encourage Expressing Emotions
   Teach kids to use words to express their feelings.
   -Benefit: Helps them process emotions and reduces tantrums and outbursts.

16. Use a Reward System for Responsibilities
   Create a chart to track chores and responsibilities.
   -Benefit: Motivates kids to help out and teaches them about accountability.

17. Plan Special "Big Kid" Activities
   Schedule outings or activities specifically for the older children.
   -Benefit: Helps them feel special and valued, reducing feelings of jealousy.

18. Keep a Well-Stocked Bag for Outings
   Prepare a bag with snacks, toys, and essentials for each child.
   -Benefit: Prevents meltdowns and ensures you're prepared for any situation.

19. Encourage Creative Play Together
   Set up art or building projects they can do as a team.
   -Benefit: Stimulates creativity and promotes collaboration.

20. Seek Support When Needed
   Don't hesitate to ask for help from family or friends.
   -Benefit: Provides extra hands and emotional support, helping you manage multiple needs more effectively.

When my kids were in the NICU, the nurses' precise schedules and routines were a lifesaver. It was like we had a blueprint for when we brought them home. But once we were on our own, it was up to me to maintain that structure. And honestly, there were times when it felt like everything was falling apart. In the beginning, it seemed like chaos reigned at least half of the time. The kids would cry, needing me at the same time, and I'd feel pulled in every direction. But I knew that if I stuck to our routines, things would eventually smooth out.

Having my husband home for the full six weeks of paternity leave with our last two was a game-changer. With our first two, he could only take a few days off, and I remember calling him in tears, overwhelmed and exhausted. He'd drop everything to come home and help, but I always felt guilty for needing him. With our last two, we got to tag-team the nights, and I wasn't alone in those hard moments. It felt like we could really manage things together, and it made a world of difference.

Even now, there are moments that feel tough. It's not perfect. But compared to those early days, it's a world of difference. What used to feel chaotic 50% of the time now feels like a rare, brief struggle—maybe 7% of the time, if I had to guess. It's amazing how quickly they grow, not just physically but mentally too. They've learned to adapt, to share, and to play together. We've gone from scrambling to manage multiple needs to watching them blossom into best friends.

Seeing them like this, it's hard to believe how overwhelming it once was. They still go through phases together—teething or growth spurts—that can throw us off. But those rough patches are fewer and farther between. Most days, our home is filled with laughter, and they play so well together that I sometimes wonder how we got here. It's a reminder that those hard days really do get easier, and that structure and support can transform chaos into something truly beautiful.

Bonding with Your Newborn

1. Skin-to-Skin Contact
   Holding your baby skin-to-skin helps regulate their body temperature and heart rate.
   -Benefit: Strengthens emotional bonding, boosts oxytocin levels, and supports breastfeeding success.

2. Eye Contact During Feeding
   Maintain eye contact while feeding your baby.
   -Benefit: Enhances emotional connection and helps with early social and visual development.

3. Gentle Touch and Massage
   Use gentle touch and massage to soothe your baby.
   -Benefit: Reduces cortisol levels (stress hormone) and promotes relaxation and sleep.

4. Reading Aloud
   Read simple, rhythmic stories to your baby.
   -Benefit: Supports early language development and creates a calming routine.

5. Talking and Singing
   Narrate your day, talk softly, or sing lullabies.
   -Benefit: Familiarizes your baby with your voice and aids in auditory and language development.

6. Babywearing
   Use a baby carrier to keep your baby close while you move around.
   -Benefit: Promotes bonding, reduces crying, and allows for hands-free movement.

7. Responding to Cries
  Quickly respond to your baby's cries to meet their needs.
  -Benefit: Builds trust and security, fostering a strong emotional
attachment.

8. Mirroring Facial Expressions
  Make and mirror simple facial expressions with your baby.
  -Benefit: Supports early social development and emotional recognition.

9. Breastfeeding or Bottle Feeding
  Use feeding times as a moment of calm connection.
  -Benefit: Enhances bonding and provides essential nutrients and
antibodies.

10. Taking Walks Together
  Go for walks with your baby in a stroller or carrier.
  -Benefit: Provides fresh air and new sensory experiences while
strengthening your connection.

11. Bath Time Bonding
  Make bath time a fun, soothing ritual.
  -Benefit: Supports sensory development and can be a calming
end-of-day activity.

12. Playful Interactions
  Engage in gentle play like peek-a-boo or making silly faces.
  -Benefit: Stimulates cognitive and emotional development and reinforces
bonding.

13. Listening to Music Together
  Play soothing music or lullabies while holding your baby.
  -Benefit: Promotes auditory development and can be calming for both
parent and child.

14. Creating a Calming Bedtime Routine
  Establish a consistent bedtime routine that includes quiet bonding activities.
  -Benefit: Helps your baby learn to self-soothe and sets the stage for healthy sleep habits.

15. Laying on the Floor Together
  Spend time laying on a soft mat or blanket on the floor, facing your baby.
  -Benefit: Encourages tummy time and strengthens the baby's neck and shoulder muscles.

16. Scent Bonding
  Keep a piece of clothing with your scent near your baby.
  -Benefit: Your scent provides comfort and security, reducing separation anxiety.

17. Encouraging Coos and Gurgles
  Respond to your baby's vocalizations with enthusiasm.
  -Benefit: Encourages communication skills and helps your baby feel heard and understood.

18. Introducing Soft Toys and Blankets
  Use soft toys or blankets for your baby to touch and explore.
  -Benefit: Provides comfort and supports tactile development.

19. Playing in Different Positions
  Hold your baby in different positions to provide varied views of the world.
  -Benefit: Helps with motor skill development and provides new perspectives for cognitive growth.

20. Mindful Parenting
  Stay present and mindful during interactions, putting away distractions like phones.
  -Benefit: Deepens the emotional connection and ensures that your baby feels valued and loved.

When my babies were born, I knew I wanted to bond with them deeply, but it wasn't always easy. I tried to cherish every small moment—taking them for walks, holding them skin-to-skin, and playing with them on the floor. I would sing songs softly and read books, their little eyes wide with curiosity. Each tiny smile or coo felt like a reward for the effort I put into connecting with them.

There were days, especially after I had postpartum depression, when it felt like I was just going through the motions. It was hard to feel that magical bond everyone talked about. The simple things, like cuddling or making silly faces, sometimes felt overwhelming. I remember sitting there, holding my baby, feeling numb, and wondering if I was doing enough.

But I kept at it. Even on the hardest days, I made sure to go for our walks, to talk and sing, even when I didn't feel like it. I reminded myself that my effort mattered, that these small, consistent actions were building a foundation. Slowly, the fog began to lift. I found myself looking forward to those quiet moments again—holding my baby close, feeling their little body relax against mine, or watching them laugh at the silly faces I made.

One of the most powerful moments was when I saw how much they responded to my voice and touch. I would read to them, pointing out pictures and making funny voices, and they would watch me so intently, little smiles forming on their lips. It made all the struggles worth it. I realized that even when I didn't feel connected, I was still laying the groundwork for a bond that would grow stronger every day.

Now, that bond is undeniable. My kids and I have an incredible connection. We have inside jokes, and they still light up when I start singing those same silly songs from when they were babies. It wasn't always easy, but staying present and putting in the effort, even when it felt hard, paid off in ways I could have never imagined. It's a bond built on countless small moments, each one a step closer to the deep, loving relationship we have now.

Chapter 5
Breastfeeding and Pumping Essentials

Managing Breastfeeding with Older Kids Around

1. Nursing Cover
Use a lightweight nursing cover that drapes over your shoulders and the baby. Choose one with an open neckline to maintain eye contact with your baby while covering yourself from view.
 - Benefit: Provides privacy, helping moms feel comfortable around older kids.

2. Nursing Pillow
 Place the pillow on your lap and position the baby on top of it, ensuring that your baby's mouth is aligned with your nipple. This keeps your arms free to manage other tasks.
 - Benefit: Offers support for the baby and reduces strain on your arms and back.

3. Designated Breastfeeding Area
Choose a comfortable chair or spot in your home, or two spots away from noise and distractions. Keep breastfeeding essentials nearby, like burp cloths, water for yourself, bottles, bottle drying rack, bottle warmer, mini fridge, diapers, wipes, extra onesies, gripe water and snacks and water for older kids.
 - Benefit: A quiet, consistent space helps avoid distractions and improves feeding focus.

4. Hands-Free Pumping Bra
 Wear a hands-free pumping bra, insert the pump flanges, and secure them. You can now pump both sides while reading to older kids or doing other light tasks.
- Benefit: Allows multitasking while pumping, freeing up your hands.

5. Snack Packs for Older Kids
Prepare snack packs (fruit, crackers, or pre-cut veggies) ahead of time and
hand them out when you start nursing. This ensures they have something
to focus on while you feed.
- Benefit: Keeps older children occupied, reducing interruptions during
feeding.

6. Educational Books About Babies
   Read simple, age-appropriate books to your children about being a big
sibling and the baby's needs. Involve them in choosing the books so they
feel engaged.
- Benefit: Helps older kids understand what's happening, reducing jealousy
and confusion.

7. Milk Storage Bags
   After pumping, pour the milk into pre-sterilized storage bags. Label each
bag with the date and amount, then store it flat in the freezer to save space
and make thawing easier.
- Benefit: Allows you to store extra milk for later use, offering flexibility.

8. Sippy Cups for Older Kids
   Prepare their favorite drink in a spill-proof sippy cup. Offer it to them when
you start feeding the baby so they can enjoy their drink while you nurse.
 - Benefit: Giving older kids a drink while breastfeeding reduces jealousy
and keeps them hydrated.

9. Baby Feeding Timer App
Download a feeding tracker app on your phone. Start the timer when you
begin feeding and track which side you nursed on, so you can manage time
between feeds and activities with your older kids.
   - Benefit: Tracks feeding times and helps you balance breastfeeding with
older kids' schedules.

10. Bottle Warmer

Pour breast milk into a bottle, place it in the bottle warmer, and heat it to the desired temperature. Teach older children how to help with this, fostering a sense of responsibility.
- Benefit: Prepares milk quickly, enabling older kids to help feed the baby.

11. Burp Rags

Keep burp rags within arm's reach during feeding. Place one over your shoulder or across the baby's chest to catch spills and minimize mess.
- Benefit: Keeps messes under control, allowing for smoother breastfeeding sessions.

12. Nursing-Friendly Clothes

Wear shirts or dresses with easy-access panels, zippers, or buttons that allow quick access for breastfeeding, reducing the time spent getting situated.
- Benefit: Makes it easy to transition between breastfeeding and caring for older children.

13. Age-Appropriate Toys

Set up a designated play area near your breastfeeding station with toys that match your older kids' age and interests. Rotate the toys regularly to keep them engaged.
- Benefit: Keeps toddlers entertained during breastfeeding, reducing interruptions.

14. Older Kids' Help With Burping

Once you've fed the baby, place the baby over your shoulder or lap and have your older child gently pat the baby's back. Supervise to make sure they are doing it safely.
- Benefit: Encourages sibling bonding and responsibility.

15. Books for Storytime During Feeding
Keep a stack of favorite books within arm's reach. Read aloud to your older child as you nurse the baby, creating a shared activity that keeps everyone engaged.
   - Benefit: Engages older kids during nursing sessions and fosters bonding.

16. Quiet Activities
Set up quiet activities like puzzles, coloring books, or crafts near your breastfeeding area. Encourage your older kids to work on these while you feed the baby.
   - Benefit: Gives older children something to focus on while you breastfeed, reducing interruptions.

17. Screen Time (in moderation)
Allow your older kids some screen time, such as watching a favorite show or playing an educational app, while you breastfeed. Set time limits and balance it with other activities.
   - Benefit: A temporary distraction that allows you to focus on feeding the baby.

18. Set Boundaries
 Have a calm conversation with your older kids about breastfeeding time. Explain that during this time, they should either play quietly or engage in a specific activity.
   - Benefit: Teaches older children when it's time to let you focus on the baby, fostering independence.

19. Sibling Feeding Time
Coordinate meal or snack times with the baby's feeding schedule. Prepare a snack or drink for your older child as you nurse or bottle-feed the baby, so they feel involved.
   - Benefit: Feeding older children during the baby's feeding time reduces sibling jealousy.

20. Praise and Positive Reinforcement
 Praise your older kids when they help or behave well during feeding times.
Positive reinforcement, like a high-five or words of encouragement, builds
confidence and encourages them to continue helping.
 - Benefit: Encourages helpful behavior from older kids and fosters sibling
bonding.

When my child was born, I realized I had to figure out how to manage
breastfeeding with two older children around. I wanted them to feel
included, not ignored, but also knew I needed time to focus on the baby. My
stepson, who was old enough to understand more about what was going
on, wanted to help out however he could. I decided to let him bottle-feed
the baby from time to time, and it became one of the most heartwarming
parts of our routine.

I would set everything up for him—make sure the bottle was ready and
prop the baby up with pillows to support his little arms. He'd sit there,
beaming with pride, holding the bottle while I supervised. It wasn't
perfect—sometimes I had to jump in to adjust the bottle or ensure the baby
wasn't getting too much air—but watching them bond made the effort
worthwhile.

The younger ones needed more help, of course. I had to guide their tiny
hands to hold the bottle just right and make sure they were sitting safely.
There were moments when I worried they might drop the bottle or tip it
over, so I stayed close, ensuring everything went smoothly.

Efficient Pumping to Stay Flexible

3. Portable Pump
Charge your portable pump fully. Strap it on, secure the flanges, and adjust
the settings for comfort. You can walk around or continue tasks while it
works quietly in the background.
   - Benefit: Keeps you mobile, allowing you to pump anywhere, even when
caring for your other children.

4. Scheduled Pumping Sessions
Set reminders on your phone to pump at regular intervals, such as every
2-3 hours. Stick to this schedule to maintain your supply and adapt it to fit
around your children's routines.
   - Benefit: Establishes a routine, ensuring consistent milk production and
predictability in your day.

5. Breast Milk Storage Bags
After pumping, pour the milk into sterilized storage bags. Seal them
properly, label with the date, and store them flat in the freezer for easy
thawing and space-saving storage.
   - Benefit: Allows you to store extra milk for future feedings, giving you
flexibility.

6. Pump Cleaning Wipes
 Keep a pack of pump cleaning wipes handy. After each pumping session,
use the wipes to quickly clean the flanges and connectors before storing
them for the next use.
   - Benefit: Cleans pump parts quickly between sessions, helping you stay
organized without needing to stop everything.

7. Pump Parts Organizer
Use a small, compartmentalized organizer for all your pump parts, including flanges, valves, and bottles. Keep this organizer near your pumping station to avoid misplaced items and quick setup.
 - Benefit: Keeps all pump accessories in one place, reducing the risk of losing parts.

8. Nursing/Pumping Tracker App
Download a breastfeeding/pumping app and log your sessions, including the amount pumped and feeding times. This helps track your supply and adjust schedules based on your baby's needs.
 - Benefit: Helps monitor milk production and manage pumping times with precision.

9. Milk Cooler Bag
Place freshly pumped milk into bottles or storage bags and keep them in an insulated cooler bag with ice packs. Use the milk within 24 hours or freeze for later.
 - Benefit: Allows you to safely store milk while on the go, ensuring you always have fresh milk for your baby.

10. Bottle Warmer
Pour breast milk into a bottle and place it in the bottle warmer. Set the warmer to the appropriate setting for breast milk, and in a few minutes, it'll be ready to feed the baby.
 - Benefit: Heats milk to the right temperature quickly, making bottle-feeding more convenient.

11. Pump Sanitizer
After washing pump parts, place them in a steam sterilizer or use a microwave sterilizing bag to eliminate germs and bacteria.
 - Benefit: Sterilizes pump parts, promoting the health of your baby and ensuring cleanliness.

12. Extra Pump Parts
Keep an extra set of pump parts on hand so that when one set is being
cleaned, you have another ready for the next session.
   - Benefit: Reduces downtime between pumping sessions, allowing you to
always have clean parts ready.

13. Pump Shields of Different Sizes
Measure your nipple size to ensure a proper fit for the flange. Having
different sizes on hand can help find the most comfortable one, preventing
pain and increasing milk output.
   - Benefit: Ensures comfort and efficient milk expression by using the right
size shields.

14. Breastfeeding-friendly Diet
Eat foods rich in proteins, healthy fats, and hydration-boosting nutrients like
oats, nuts, leafy greens, and plenty of water throughout the day.
   - Benefit: Supports milk production and gives you the energy you need to
care for your baby and older children.

15. Hydration
Drink at least 8 glasses of water daily, and keep a water bottle near your
pumping or breastfeeding area to remind you to hydrate while feeding or
pumping.
   - Benefit: Staying hydrated is essential to maintaining a steady milk
supply.

16. Quiet Pump
Choose a pump that is known for being quiet, and set it up in a comfortable
spot where you won't disturb anyone. Use it when the household is calmer
or during nap times for minimal interruption.
   - Benefit: Reduces noise, making it easier to pump discreetly without
disturbing your children or the baby during naps.

17. Power Bank
Charge a portable power bank and connect your pump to it when you're on the move or don't have access to electricity. This is especially handy for travel or being outdoors with the kids.
   - Benefit: Keeps your pump running when there's no access to an outlet, ensuring you never miss a session.

18. Nursing-Friendly Tops
Wear nursing tops with hidden panels or quick-access zippers, buttons, or pull-down fabric. This saves time and makes the process smoother, especially when you have other kids needing attention.
   - Benefit: Allows you to easily switch between breastfeeding and pumping with minimal effort.

19. Pump Bag
Invest in a pump bag that has compartments for your pump, bottles, cords, and flanges. Use it to carry everything you need when you leave the house or move between rooms at home. This way, you always have your pump setup organized and ready.
   - Benefit: Makes it easy to transport your pump and accessories wherever you go.

20. Support System
Build a support system by involving your partner, family, or friends. They can help with household chores or taking care of your older kids while you focus on pumping or breastfeeding. Don't hesitate to ask for help when you need it, especially in those early, exhausting weeks.
   - Benefit: Ensures you have emotional and practical help during breastfeeding and pumping, reducing stress.

After my second child was born, I realized that pumping would be essential to maintaining some semblance of freedom and flexibility, especially with older kids to take care of. There were so many moments when I was chasing a toddler, trying to soothe a baby, and pumping all at once! I quickly learned that hands-free pumping was a lifesaver.

By having a routine, I could pump without feeling overwhelmed, and with older kids around, it gave me the chance to still be present with them. They even found it fascinating and loved helping me put the milk away in the freezer.

When I was in the thick of those early days with my newborn, I had my setup next to my bed so finely tuned that it felt like a well-oiled machine. On the nightstand, there were burp cloths always within reach, water for myself (because hydration was key), bottles ready for the baby, and a drying rack for when I washed them. The bottle warmer sat there, easy to grab, along with a mini fridge stocked with milk. I kept extra onesies, diapers, and wipes all lined up, and even a bottle of gripe water in case it was needed.

During the day when my husband was home, it became a little routine. I'd tag out with the older kids, sending them off for a snack or an activity, and go to my quiet corner of the room. This was my time to pump, feed the baby, and bond with them. I'd grab a snack, maybe something quick to eat, and just focus on them, taking in the calm of those moments before jumping back into the whirlwind of a busy home. It was like a mini-break, despite the hustle around me.

Sometimes, we had company over, and I'd see it as the perfect excuse to sneak away for a moment of solitude. I'd hand the baby off to my husband or a guest, give them a bottle, and quietly slip away with my pump. Of course, only if my husband was around to supervise, I needed to make sure the baby was in good hands while I took a moment for myself.

If my husband wasn't home, I'd have to get creative. I'd set myself up with my hands-free pump, which gave me the freedom to move around, and make sure the older kids were set up with their food or a snack, something to drink to keep them occupied. It wasn't always the most relaxing pumping session, but it was necessary. And somehow, in the middle of all that chaos, I still found peace in knowing I was giving my baby what they needed, while also taking care of myself.

Navigating Supply and Demand with Multiple Little Ones

1. Feed/Pump on Schedule
Create a feeding and pumping schedule that works with your baby's natural rhythms.Aim to feed or pump every 2-3 hours during the day for newborns and every 3-4 hours as they grow.Use a hands-free pumping bra to make the process easier and more comfortable while multitasking.Track your milk output to monitor your supply and make adjustments as needed.
-Benefit:Helps establish and maintain a steady milk supply.Reduces the likelihood of engorgement or mastitis.Encourages your baby to feed efficiently and regularly, which supports their growth and development.

2. Supplement with Pumped Milk
Pump during sessions on both sides or one and store milk. Use it for bottle feeds when you need a break or someone else needs to take over while you attend to your older kids.
   - Benefit: Ensures no feeding time is missed even if you're busy with your other kids.

3.Make Breast Milk Soap
Save any extra or unused breast milk that is past its expiration for soap making.Use a soap-making kit or ingredients such as lye, coconut oil, olive oil, and your breast milk.Carefully follow soap-making instructions, as working with lye requires safety precautions.Let the soap cure for several weeks before use.
-Benefit:Breast milk contains natural moisturizers, antioxidants, and nutrients like vitamin A, which can nourish and hydrate the skin.Using breast milk in soap may help with conditions like eczema or dry skin.It's a way to repurpose extra milk that may have been thrown away, reducing waste.

4. Hydrate Often
Keep a water bottle with you at all times, especially during nursing sessions. Aim for about 8-10 glasses of water a day to support milk production.
  - Benefit: Staying hydrated is essential for maintaining milk production.

5. Eat Nutrient-Dense Foods
Include foods rich in protein, healthy fats, and complex carbs like nuts, whole grains, and leafy greens in your daily meals.
  - Benefit: Provides your body with the essential nutrients needed for milk production.

6. Rest When You Can
Nap when your baby naps, and delegate chores or child care when possible to prioritize sleep, even if it's in small increments.
  - Benefit: Helps prevent fatigue, which can negatively affect your milk supply.

7. Babywearing for Hands-Free Nursing
Use a baby carrier or sling that allows for nursing on the go. Adjust the carrier so that the baby can comfortably nurse while you walk around or engage with your older children.
  - Benefit: Allows you to nurse while keeping your hands free to care for older kids.

8. Use Lactation Supplements
Try fenugreek, brewer's yeast, or oatmeal-based supplements. Always consult your healthcare provider before starting supplements to ensure they are safe for you.
  - Benefit: Helps increase milk supply when needed.

9. Alternate Feeding Positions
Change up your feeding positions—cradle hold, football hold, or side-lying—to help empty different areas of the breast and keep milk flowing efficiently.
  - Benefit: Prevents blocked ducts and ensures even milk flow.

10.Consider Formula
If you're supplementing with formula, choose a product appropriate for your baby's age and needs (e.g., infant formula for the first 6 months).Follow the formula's instructions carefully for preparation, including water-to-powder ratio.Gradually introduce formula alongside breast milk to help your baby adjust, especially if transitioning from breast milk.
-Benefit:Formula is a reliable source of nutrients and can be essential for parents who are unable to breastfeed exclusively.Provides convenience, especially when you're away or need a break from direct breastfeeding.Formula-fed babies often sleep longer, due to the slower digestion of formula compared to breast milk.

11. Use Different Pumping Methods
Alternate between hands-free and manual pumping to adapt to your needs throughout the day. Having both options ready can increase supply while allowing flexibility when you're caring for multiple kids.
-Benefits: Increases milk production and lets you multitask, freeing up time to care for your other children.

12. Skin-to-Skin Contact
Hold your baby skin-to-skin before or during feedings. Simply lay your baby on your chest with only a diaper, and cover with a blanket for warmth. This promotes the release of oxytocin, which boosts milk supply.   - Benefit: Encourages bonding and stimulates milk production.

13. Pumping After and during Feedings
After and during each feeding session, pump for an additional 5-10
minutes. This empties the breasts further and encourages your body to
produce more milk.
   - Benefit: Helps signal your body to produce more milk.

14. Monitor Wet Diapers
Count the wet diapers—6-8 wet diapers per day usually indicates that the
baby is getting enough milk.
   - Benefit: Ensures your baby is getting enough milk.

15. Burp, Then Try to Feed More
Burp your baby after each 1-2 ounces of feeding, especially during bottle
feeding.Try to feed again after burping, as burping can sometimes relieve
discomfort or gas, making room for more milk.
-Benefit:Reduces the likelihood of discomfort from trapped air in the
stomach.Encourages better digestion and reduces spit-up.Aids in creating
a peaceful feeding experience for both you and your baby.

16. Educate Yourself on How Much Your Baby Should Be Eating at Their
Age
Research age-appropriate feeding amounts. For instance, newborns
typically eat 1-3 ounces every 2-3 hours. As babies grow, their intake
increases to about 4-6 ounces per feed at 1 month and 6-8 ounces per
feed by 3 months.Monitor your baby's growth by checking in with their
pediatrician and tracking their feeding habits.Offer more milk if your baby is
still showing signs of hunger after burping and finishing their bottle.
-Benefit:Educating yourself ensures that you are meeting your baby's
nutritional needs.Helps establish a routine that supports healthy growth and
development.Provides peace of mind, knowing you are feeding your baby
according to expert guidelines.

17. Involve Older Kids in Feeding Time
Allow older kids to help by handing you a burp cloth, picking out a book to
read to the baby, or sitting with you during feeding.
   - Benefit: Reduces interruptions and jealousy.

18. Reduce Stress
Practice self-care—take deep breaths, meditate, or ask for help when
needed. Reducing stress can directly improve milk production.
   - Benefit: Stress can negatively affect milk production.

19. Cup of Milk for Older Kids
When you sit down to nurse, give your older child their own cup of milk or
water. This helps them mimic the baby and feel part of the process.
   - Benefit: Helps older children feel included while you're nursing.

20. Praise Older Kids for Patience
Praise your older child when they wait patiently or help during feeding. You
can say, "Thank you for being so helpful and patient," to encourage
continued good behavior.
   - Benefit: Reinforces positive behavior during feeding times.

As time went on, I started noticing a change in my stepson's behavior. He had been so excited about the baby's arrival, but now that the baby was here, he was feeling a bit left out. His playful energy started to turn into frustration whenever I had to nurse the baby, and I could sense a growing jealousy. Eventually, I decided we needed help, so we went to see a therapist. The therapist gave us some excellent advice that seemed almost too simple: "When you feed the baby, give your older child something to do that mimics the baby's actions. If the baby is drinking milk, offer your older child their own drink—something like a cup of milk or water."

It was worth a try, so I put the plan into action. The next time I sat down to nurse the baby, I handed my stepson a cup of milk and told him that while the baby was eating, he could have a snack too. To my surprise, it worked almost immediately. He didn't seem jealous anymore. Instead, he would sit beside me, quietly sipping his milk, feeling like he was part of the routine. I saw a complete change in his demeanor, as if that small gesture made him feel just as important.

The breastfeeding journey was one I had to manage with precision and creativity. I remember the days when I would put the baby on one breast and attach the pump to the other. It was a balancing act, but it worked—keeping everything even as I pumped while breastfeeding. Sometimes, I would go all in and bottle-feed while pumping both breasts at the same time. The result was incredible—I was producing so much milk that it felt like an achievement, like my body was truly working in sync with my baby's needs. There was something so relieving about emptying out both sides, a weight lifting off my chest, literally.

Interestingly, the sound of the pump's rhythmic whir was soothing for my baby. Sometimes, they'd even drift off to sleep while feeding. But that wasn't exactly what I wanted. I needed them to stay awake and feed well so they'd be full enough to nap after. So, I'd gently rub their cheek or pull the bottle out a little to prompt them to keep drinking. If they were dozing off, I'd carefully burp them, just to get them to take a few more sips, and it worked. It felt like a little victory each time, ensuring they had enough before they rested.

Two of my kids had sensitive stomachs, so burping was an essential part of every feeding. It wasn't just about the bottles or the breast; it was about making sure they weren't uncomfortable. I'd do tummy rubs, bicycle legs, and knee tucks—little techniques I'd learned that helped relieve their gas and discomfort. It wasn't always easy, but it was worth it. And when I eventually switched to a sensitive formula for them, I noticed a huge improvement in their stomachs. It was a relief.

Despite the switch to formula, I continued pumping. It was a part of my routine that had become both a necessity and a release. Not only did it ease the discomfort in my breasts, but I also found a way to repurpose the milk, making breast milk soap for a soothing, natural skin treatment. Over time, I gradually tapered off. I tried to just stop pumping completely at one point, but my body didn't want to cooperate. My breasts felt like they were going to explode, full to the brim with milk that needed to be released. It was a painful reminder of how much I'd been giving, how hard my body had worked to provide, and how hard it was to let go.

It was a journey of dedication, figuring out how to balance everything, even the discomforts, for the sake of my baby and my body. Eventually, I found peace in knowing I had given my all and that, even as I slowly stepped away, I'd always have that bond.

Chapter 6
Sleep Training for Different Ages

Creating a Routine that Works for All Kids

1. Set a Consistent Bedtime
Pick a bedtime and stick to it every night for all kids.
-Benefit: Helps regulate their internal clocks and makes winding down easier.

2. Create a Wind-Down Ritual
Use calming activities like bath time, storytime, or lullabies before bed.
-Benefit: Prepares them mentally and physically for sleep.

3. Dim the Lights
Lower lighting an hour before bed to create a calm environment.
-Benefit: Promotes melatonin production to aid in sleep.

4. Use White Noise or Calming Music
Play soft white noise or relaxing music to help soothe all children.
-Benefit: Drowns out household noise and creates a peaceful sleep environment.

5. Keep Bedtime Items Consistent
Use familiar items like favorite blankets, stuffed animals, or specific pajamas.
-Benefit: Provides comfort and security, making it easier for them to settle down.

6. Have Synchronized Nap Times
Have all younger kids nap at the same time, and allow older children to have quiet time with activities or homeschooling.
-Benefit: Helps maintain routine and allows for productive time with older kids or self-care.

7. Create a Quiet Time Before Bed
Spend 30 minutes on quiet activities like puzzles or reading.
-Benefit: Reduces stimulation, helping kids transition to bedtime.

8. Limit Screen Time Before Bed
Stop screen time at least an hour before bed.
-Benefit: Prevents overstimulation and encourages melatonin production.

9. Ensure Comfortable Sleeping Spaces
Make sure each child's sleeping area is quiet, cozy, and suited to their needs.
-Benefit: A comfortable sleep environment promotes restful sleep.

10. Use a Timer for Transitions
Set a timer to signal when it's almost bedtime.
-Benefit: Helps kids mentally prepare and avoids last-minute surprises.

11. Incorporate Bedtime Stories
Read a short, calming story to each child or as a group.
-Benefit: Strengthens family bonds and provides a relaxing wind-down activity.

12. Offer a Security Object
Provide a small blanket or stuffed animal to help them feel safe.
-Benefit: Helps children self-soothe during the night.

13. Use a Nightlight for Toddlers
Place a soft night light in the room for kids who fear the dark.
-Benefit: Offers reassurance without disturbing their sleep.

14. Introduce a Sleep Chart for Older Kids
Use a chart to reward older children for staying in bed all night.
-Benefit: Encourages responsibility and adds a fun element to bedtime.

15. Offer a Light Snack Before Bed
Give a small snack, like crackers or fruit, avoiding sugary treats.
-Benefit: Prevents hunger-related sleep disruptions.

16. Create a Calm Evening Environment
Keep the household calm in the hours leading up to bedtime.
-Benefit: Helps set a peaceful mood, making it easier for kids to settle
down.

17. Use the "One More Time" Rule
Limit requests for water, stories, or bathroom trips to one before bed.
-Benefit: Avoids unnecessary delays and helps kids settle into sleep faster.

18. Be Consistent and Patient
Stick to your routine, even if some nights are tough. Adjust as needed, but
remain steady.
-Benefit: Children thrive on consistency, and sticking to a routine will lead to
long-term success.

19. Include Quiet Time During the Day
Schedule quiet time during the day, especially for toddlers.
-Benefit: Helps prevent them from becoming overtired, which can lead to
bedtime resistance.

20. Monitor Room Temperature
Ensure the room stays between 68-72°F for optimal sleep conditions.
-Benefit: A comfortable environment prevents sleep disruptions due to
discomfort.

Synchronizing my children's naps quickly became a non-negotiable in our daily routine. With multiple little ones so close in age, that nap time turned into a golden window where I could actually get things done—whether it was tidying up, prepping meals, or even just taking a quiet moment to myself. It was a time I could count on, knowing the house would be peaceful for a couple of hours.

But as my older two grew, they stopped napping around the age of four. That shift could have been chaotic, but instead, it became a precious opportunity. During those quiet afternoon hours when the younger ones napped, I started homeschooling the older two. It was perfect—I could give them my full attention without the distraction of the babies, and we could dive into learning together. The routine evolved naturally, and I cherished that dedicated time to focus on them while their younger siblings rested.

Another lifesaver in our sleep routine has been security objects. Each of my kids has something they're deeply attached to—a special blanket, a toy, something that gives them comfort and helps them fall asleep. These objects are like magic when it comes to soothing them, whether it's getting to sleep initially, settling back down if they wake up or when they are sick. And if we're out and about, having that object on hand can make all the difference.

Of course, there's a downside—if anything happens to that treasured item, it can quickly turn into a no-fun situation. We've had a few moments of panic when something went missing or got damaged, and after that, I wised up. Now, the moment I notice one of my kids getting attached to something, I immediately buy two. One stays tucked away in the closet, just in case. If it's a toy with batteries, I take them out of the backup, so when it's time to switch, I'm not dealing with a gross, corroded mess. Having that extra on hand has saved me so many times, and it's one of those tricks I wish I'd known from the start!
It's funny how something so small like a nap routine or a security object can make such a big difference in managing the chaos of daily life with multiple little ones.

Sleep Training Techniques for the Newborn

1. Set Up a Routine
Establish consistent bedtimes and nap times to help your newborn recognize sleep cues.
-Benefit: Helps regulate your baby's internal clock and promotes better sleep quality.

2. Swaddling
Wrap your baby snugly in a swaddle to mimic the womb.
Benefit: Reduces startle reflex, allowing longer, more restful sleep.

3. Create a Soothing Sleep Environment
Keep the room dim, quiet, and at a comfortable temperature.
-Benefit: Promotes a calm environment conducive to sleep, reducing overstimulation.

4. White Noise or Soft Music
Play gentle sounds or white noise to mask background noise.
-Benefit: Helps soothe the baby and blocks out disruptive sounds, aiding in longer sleep stretches.

5. Full Tummy Before Bed
Feed your baby before putting them down to sleep to ensure they aren't hungry.
-Benefit: A well-fed baby is more likely to sleep longer between feedings.

6. Set Up a Baby Monitor or Camera
Use a baby monitor with a camera to check on your newborn without entering the room.
-Benefit: Allows you to monitor their sleep without interruptions, which can prevent unnecessary wake-ups.

7. Gradual Sleep Training
Slowly increase the time between soothing your baby when they cry to
teach them self-soothing techniques.
-Benefit: Helps your baby learn to fall asleep on their own, leading to more
independent sleep over time.

8. Consistency with Wake-Up Time
Wake your baby up at the same time every day, even if they wake up at
night.
-Benefit: Reinforces their natural circadian rhythm and helps create a
predictable schedule.

9. Use a Nighttime Routine
Include a bath, story, or lullaby in the evening to signal bedtime.
-Benefit: Helps the baby wind down and understand it's time for sleep.

10. Dim Lights Before Bedtime
Lower the lights about 30 minutes before sleep.
-Benefit: Encourages melatonin production, which helps your baby fall
asleep faster.

11. Offer a Comfort Item
Once your baby is old enough, introduce a soft blanket or stuffed animal.
-Benefit: Provides comfort and security, making it easier for them to fall
asleep on their own.

12. Avoid Overtiredness
Watch for signs of tiredness, like rubbing eyes or yawning, and put your
baby to sleep before they get overtired.
-Benefit: Prevents fussiness and helps them fall asleep easier.

13. Sleep in Short Bursts During the Day
Encourage naps throughout the day, but don't let them nap too long before
bedtime.
-Benefit: Daytime naps prevent overtiredness and help nighttime sleep
come more easily.

14. Lay Down While Drowsy but Awake
Place your baby in their crib when they are sleepy but still awake.
-Benefit: Teaches them to fall asleep independently, without needing to be
rocked or fed to sleep.

15. Offer Pacifiers (If Appropriate)
Provide a pacifier to soothe your baby to sleep.
-Benefit: May help reduce the risk of SIDS and provides comfort.

16. Gentle Sleep Cues
Use calming techniques, such as patting or shushing, instead of picking
your baby up immediately when they wake.
-Benefit: Helps the baby learn to self-soothe without relying on external
comfort.

17. Stick to Nap Times
Ensure naps happen at consistent times each day, in the same sleep
environment.
-Benefit: Builds a reliable daily rhythm and improves nighttime sleep.

18. Comfortable Crib Setup
Use a firm mattress with a fitted sheet and avoid blankets or pillows for safe
sleep.
-Benefit: Encourages safe and comfortable sleep while reducing the risk of
SIDS.

19. Track Sleep Patterns
Keep a log of sleep patterns to identify what's working or when adjustments
need to be made.
-Benefit: Provides insights into your baby's routine, allowing for better
planning.

20. Patience and Flexibility
Understand that each baby's sleep pattern evolves, so be patient and
flexible with sleep training.
-Benefit: Reduces stress on parents and baby by allowing room for growth
and change.

When my first baby was born, I quickly got used to those first couple of
weeks when they seemed to sleep all the time. It's easy to think, "This isn't
so bad!" But as time passed, I realized that without a schedule, I was
setting myself up for disaster. I had heard so many people say it wasn't
possible to get a newborn on a routine, so I didn't even try at first.

Then, one day, I met a nurse who changed everything. She had just had
her fifth baby, and when she mentioned that her newborn was already
sleeping through the night, I was in shock. She told me that sleep training is
absolutely possible from birth—you just have to commit to it and stay
consistent. That was the moment everything clicked for me, and I became
determined to make it work.

With my last three babies, they were all sleeping through the night by one
month old. But even before that milestone, they were on a well-tuned
schedule. Their bodies knew the routine, and so did mine. It was so much
easier knowing what to expect each day, and it brought a sense of calm to
our household that was invaluable.

Having that schedule didn't just help me, though—it made it much easier
for anyone else stepping in to help. Whether it was family or friends, they
didn't have to guess if the baby was hungry, tired, or fussy. All they had to
do was follow the schedule, and it worked like a charm.

The way I built that schedule was by carefully following my babies' natural
sleep and feeding patterns and researching how much sleep they needed
for their age. As they grew, the times changed, but I always transitioned
gradually, typically over a week. It was an adjustment, but by sticking to the
routine and making small changes over time, everything stayed smooth,
and my babies always seemed to thrive on that predictability.

I've come to realize that those early days of sticking to a routine make all
the difference in the long run, for both the baby and for me.

Managing Sleep Regressions with Other Toddlers

1. Maintain a Consistent Bedtime Routine
Stick to the same bedtime activities each night, like bath, story, and cuddles.
-Benefit: Reinforces sleep cues and helps toddlers feel secure despite changes.

2. Offer Extra Comfort
During a regression, offer additional soothing like extra cuddles or soft words.
-Benefit: Helps ease anxiety or separation fears, making it easier for the toddler to fall asleep.

3. Limit Screen Time Before Bed
Avoid screens at least an hour before sleep to prevent overstimulation.
-Benefit: Encourages melatonin production, which aids in falling asleep faster.

4. Introduce Calming Bedtime Rituals
Add new calming activities like soft music or a gentle back rub before sleep.
-Benefit: Helps your toddler relax and signals it's time for rest.

5. Keep Nap Times Consistent
Stick to regular nap times even if night sleep is disrupted.
-Benefit: Prevents overtiredness, which can worsen sleep regressions.

6. Set Boundaries with Compassion
Be firm but gentle when setting limits around bedtime (e.g., staying in bed).
-Benefit: Provides structure while addressing the child's emotional needs.

7. Sleep Environment Adjustments
Ensure your toddler's room is dark, quiet, and comfortable. Use a nightlight
if they're scared of the dark.
-Benefit: Creates a peaceful environment that promotes uninterrupted
sleep.

8. Offer a Comfort Object
Let your toddler sleep with a favorite stuffed animal or blanket.
-Benefit: Provides security and comfort, especially during a regression
phase.

9. Increase Daytime Activity
Encourage more physical play and engagement during the day.
-Benefit: Helps toddlers burn energy, leading to better sleep at night.

10. Offer a Simple Explanation
If your toddler is old enough, explain what's happening (e.g., "It's time for
sleep now").
-Benefit: Helps them understand the importance of sleep and what's
expected.

11. Gentle Reassurance When Waking
If your toddler wakes at night, offer quick and calm reassurance without
prolonged engagement.
-Benefit: Teaches them it's okay to wake but also that nighttime is for
sleeping.

12. Gradual Adjustments for Sleep Timing
If your toddler struggles to sleep at their usual time, adjust bedtime by
10-15 minutes over several days.
-Benefit: Prevents overtiredness and can help reset their internal clock.

13. Avoid Negative Sleep Associations
Try not to introduce new habits like rocking to sleep that may be hard to break.
-Benefit: Encourages long-term self-soothing without needing external aids.

14. Prioritize Daytime Nutrition
Make sure your toddler has regular meals and snacks during the day.
-Benefit: Ensures they aren't waking from hunger during sleep regressions.

15. Encourage Quiet Time if Naps are Skipped
If your toddler resists naps, offer quiet activities instead.
-Benefit: Provides rest without overtiredness, easing night-time sleep.

16. Offer a Nighttime Drink (Water)
Provide a sippy cup of water near the bed for thirst.
-Benefit: Avoids night time wake-ups due to thirst without breaking sleep with food.

17. Patience During Transitions
Regressions often coincide with milestones (e.g., potty training). Be patient and flexible with changes.
-Benefit: Reduces stress and helps toddlers feel supported during new developmental stages.

18. Limit Sugar and Stimulants Late in the Day
Avoid sugary snacks and beverages close to bedtime.
-Benefit: Prevents hyperactivity and helps wind down for restful sleep.

19. Use a Toddler Sleep Chart
Create a simple sleep chart or sticker system to encourage positive sleep habits.
-Benefit: Makes bedtime fun and gives the toddler a sense of accomplishment.

20. Stay Consistent with Discipline
If your toddler gets out of bed, calmly walk them back without extended conversation.
-Benefit: Reinforces the expectation of staying in bed without increasing attention-seeking behavior.

When my toddlers transitioned from their cribs to beds, sleep regression hit us hard. The newfound freedom of being able to get in and out of bed whenever they wanted made bedtime a lot more challenging. I had a lot to do to help them adjust to this new setup, and patience became my best friend.

At first, I'd tuck them in, sit by their bed, and reassure them it was time for sleep. Of course, being toddlers, they'd pop right back up. Every time they got out of bed, I'd calmly ask them to go back and tuck them in if needed. This became a bit of a routine itself—tucking them in, standing by the door, and repeating the process when they tried to get up again.

Eventually I moved to the next step by switching to the baby monitor with a camera. I'd sit just outside their room, and if they started to stir or get up, I'd ask them through the camera to go back to bed. It became kind of a game where they knew I was watching, but they also knew what was expected. After a while, I didn't need the camera much anymore—only on rare occasions when they were having an off night.

Sticking to a routine through all of this helped tremendously. I could see how much it affected their ability to settle in for sleep when we stayed consistent. I also noticed that on days when they skipped their nap, it threw them off. When they missed a nap, it felt like their little brains were going a million miles an hour. I'd get the sense they were on the verge of some new skill or breakthrough, like their minds were working overtime to process something we'd been practicing. Sure enough, the next day, they'd often show off a new skill—whether it was a word they'd been trying to say, figuring out a puzzle, or some other milestone.

Those napless days were tough, but once they hit that breakthrough, it was usually a one-time thing, and they'd get right back on schedule. Managing sleep regressions took a lot of patience and creativity, but it always paid off in the end.

Chapter 7
Teething

Facts about teething

1. Typical Teething Age – Most babies begin teething between 4 and 7 months, but it can start as early as 3 months or as late as 12 months.

2. First Teeth to Emerge – The lower front teeth, also called central incisors, are usually the first to come in.

3. Early Signs of Teething – Drooling, irritability, and the urge to chew on things are common early signs that teething has begun.

4. Drooling – Teething stimulates saliva production, often leading to excessive drooling, which can cause rashes around the mouth and chin.

5. Teething Rashes – The constant drool can irritate the skin around the mouth, chin, and neck, leading to red, dry patches or rashes.

6. Fever – Some babies may develop a low-grade fever during teething, but a high fever is not typical and may indicate illness.

7. Chewing Everything – Babies often soothe their sore gums by chewing on fingers, toys, or anything they can get into their mouths.

8. Swollen Gums – You may notice swollen or tender gums where the tooth is about to break through.

9. Changes in Bowel Movements – Some babies experience changes in their stool during teething, such as looser or more frequent bowel movements.

10. Disturbed Sleep – Teething pain can disrupt a baby's usual sleep patterns, causing frequent nighttime waking.

11. Increased Fussiness – As teeth push through the gums, babies often become more irritable and fussy than usual.

12. Ear Pulling – Babies sometimes pull or tug on their ears while teething, as the pain can radiate from the gums to the ears.

13. Loss of Appetite – Babies may refuse food or breast milk due to the discomfort of sore gums.

14. Sucking for Comfort – While some babies refuse to feed, others may want to nurse or suck more for comfort during teething.

15. Diaper Rash – The increase in drool and changes in bowel movements can sometimes lead to more frequent diaper rashes.

16. Tooth Eruption Timing – It can take anywhere from several days to a few weeks for a tooth to fully emerge once teething symptoms start.

17. Number of Teeth in the First Year – Most babies have about four to six teeth by their first birthday.

18. Teething in stages – Molars may begin pushing through the gums, then stop for a period of time before resuming. This process happens because the teeth are slowly working their way up, and sometimes they pause before fully emerging. The baby may experience discomfort even though the tooth is not yet visible.

19. Increased Biting – Babies may bite down on anything, even during breastfeeding, as they try to relieve gum discomfort.

20. Teething overlap–When children of different ages experience teething at the same time. This happens because teething is a developmental milestone that doesn't always follow a strict timeline, so it's possible for

siblings, even with age differences, to go through teething stages simultaneously.

My two sets of kids, just 11 months apart, always seemed to time their teething together. It felt like their molars had a mind of their own, playing a stop-and-go game that kept me guessing. One day they'd be fussing, drooling, and chewing on anything within reach, and I'd brace myself for the inevitable eruption of teeth—only for things to suddenly calm down without a tooth in sight.

At first, with my eldest, I couldn't figure it out. I would second-guess myself constantly, thinking, "Is she teething, or is something else going on?" One day she'd show all the classic signs—red cheeks, drool, the whole teething drama—and the next day, she was perfectly content, with no new teeth to blame. It wasn't until I hit the books that I learned about teething in stages. Teeth don't just pop through all at once; they shift, pause, and start again, dragging out the process for weeks or even months.

When both kids started teething at the same time, it was hard. The crying, the sleepless nights, and the endless soothing felt overwhelming at times. But in a strange way, I'm grateful it happened together. We'd have "cuddle teething days," where I'd scoop them both up, snuggle them in close, and we'd ride out the rough patches together. Those days were tough, but they also gave me a chance to slow down and be there for both of them in their discomfort.

Eventually, the molars would finally break through, and just like that, it was done. We'd move on, and I'd remind myself that even the toughest stages are only temporary.

Signs and cues of teething

1. Excessive Drooling – Increased saliva production is one of the most common signs of teething.

2. Chewing on Everything – Babies will try to chew on anything they can get their hands on to soothe their sore gums.

3. Irritability and Fussiness – Babies may become more cranky or fussy due to the discomfort of teeth pushing through the gums.

4. Red or Swollen Gums – You may notice your baby's gums look red, swollen, or even bruised as a tooth gets closer to breaking through.

5. More Cuddly – Babies might become more clingy and seek extra comfort from parents during this uncomfortable time.

6. Frequent Night Waking – Teething can disrupt sleep patterns, leading to more frequent wake-ups at night.

7. Pulling on Ears – Babies may pull at their ears as the pain from teething can radiate to the ear area.

8. Rubbing Their Cheeks – Your baby might rub their cheeks or face as a reaction to the pain from teething.

9. Decreased Appetite – Sore gums can make it uncomfortable for babies to eat, leading to reduced interest in food or breastmilk.

10. Sucking for Comfort – Some babies may want to nurse more often to comfort themselves while teething.

11. Refusing to Eat – On the other hand, some babies might refuse to eat due to the pain.

12. Low-Grade Fever – While not every baby will experience this, some may have a slight increase in body temperature during teething.

13. Crying Spells – Random, unexplained bouts of crying can be a sign of teething pain.

14. Loose or More Frequent Stools – Teething may cause changes in bowel movements for some babies, often leading to looser stools.

15. Diaper Rash – Increased drooling and changes in stools during teething can lead to diaper rash.

16. Biting More – Babies tend to bite down on objects (and sometimes even people) to relieve the discomfort of their gums.

17. Drool Rash – You may notice a rash or red patches around your baby's mouth, chin, or neck due to excessive drooling.

18. Gum Rubbing – Babies may rub their gums with their fingers or toys to alleviate discomfort.

19. Restlessness – Your baby might seem more restless and unable to settle, both during naps and at night.

20. Swollen Cheeks – Some babies will develop slightly puffy or swollen cheeks on the side where a tooth is about to emerge.

These signs can help you identify when your baby is teething, but every baby is different. Always trust your instincts and consult with your doctor if something seems off.

Each of my kids had their own unique way of showing they were teething, but after going through it with all of them, I developed a sixth sense for it. Even though their symptoms varied, they all tended to get their first teeth around the same age, and there's nothing quite like those tiny first teeth—they're just the cutest.

My third child, though, was the toughest one to figure out. She had such a determined spirit, always wanting to keep up with her older siblings, no matter what. But when those teeth started coming in, she'd do something that was completely out of character—she'd actually grab her blankie and cuddle with me. It was our little moment together.

Then there's my youngest son. Normally, he's a great sleeper, but when he's teething or hitting a growth spurt, the middle of the night becomes a whole different story. During the day, he's as tough as nails, but as soon as he lies down at night, the pain seems to catch up with him. He tends to wake up more, and I know those nighttime battles are because he's focused on the discomfort. Two things I've noticed are that he'll press his cheek into the mattress, like he's trying to find relief, and he'll wake up whining but still rubbing his gums with his fingers.

The scariest part of teething for all my kids has been the fevers. With everything happening during COVID, I was always extra cautious, but luckily for me, it was never more than a low-grade fever. Still, it was enough to keep me on my toes.

By the time each of them started teething, I felt like we had such a strong bond that I just knew. I could sense something was off before the teeth ever appeared. Sometimes, though, I wasn't sure if it was teething or growing pains. So, I'd wash my hands and gently rub around their gums or even their little legs. If I hit the right spot, they'd calm down, and I knew I was onto something. It became my way of tuning into them, knowing where to monitor and help them get through the worst of it.

Soothe your teething baby

1. Cold Teething Ring – Offer a refrigerated teething ring (not frozen) to help numb sore gums and provide relief.

2. Teething Tabs – Use homeopathic teething tablets (as recommended by your pediatrician) to help soothe discomfort.

3. Gum Massage – Gently rub your baby's gums with a clean finger to relieve pressure and pain.

4. Cold Washcloth – Wet a washcloth, refrigerate it, and let your baby chew on it to soothe their gums.

5. Breastfeeding – Nursing can offer comfort and distraction from teething pain, though some babies may bite, so be cautious.

6. Frozen Breast Milk Pops – Freeze small portions of breast milk in ice cube trays or mesh feeders to soothe sore gums.

7. Teething Gel – Use a doctor-recommended teething gel (sparingly) to numb your baby's gums.

8. Teething Biscuits – Offer teething biscuits or crackers for your baby to chew on, but supervise closely to avoid choking.

9. Cold Spoons – Place a spoon in the refrigerator and let your baby chew on the cool, smooth surface.

10. Distraction – Distract your baby with toys, music, or playtime to take their mind off teething pain.

11. Cuddle Time – Offer extra cuddles and comfort as your baby may be more clingy during teething.

12. Teething Necklace (For Parents) – Wear a silicone teething necklace for your baby to safely chew on while being held.

13. Pacifiers – Some babies find comfort in sucking on a pacifier, which can also provide relief to sore gums.

14. Chilled Fruits – If your baby has started solids, offer chilled fruit like cold slices of cucumber or watermelon in a mesh feeder.

15. Teething Mittens – Let your baby wear soft, chewable teething mittens designed for them to gnaw on safely.

16. Pain Relief Medication – If recommended by your doctor, offer baby-safe pain relievers like acetaminophen or ibuprofen to ease teething pain.

17. Teething Toys – Provide soft, silicone, toothbrush, or rubber teething toys designed for chewing to relieve discomfort.

18. Cool Water – Offer small sips of cool water (if your baby is old enough) to help soothe the gums and hydrate.

19. Keep the Area Dry – Gently pat around your baby's mouth to prevent drool rashes and discomfort caused by excessive drooling.

20. White Noise or Calming Music – Help your baby relax and sleep by playing white noise or soothing lullabies, especially if teething disrupts their sleep.

When my kids were teething, I quickly learned that each one needed a different approach to find relief. I'd start by giving them a gum massage, gently rubbing their gums to figure out exactly where the pain was coming from. Once I pinpointed the sore spot, I'd turn to teething tablets. But instead of just giving them the tablet, I would mix it with a tiny bit of water to make a paste. That way, I could apply it directly to the area causing them pain, and it worked wonders for quick relief.

Frozen teething toys were another lifesaver. The kids loved the cold sensation, but when they were really young, they'd cry because the toys were too cold to hold. I'd help them grip it until they got bigger, and then I found ones that had a handle with only one frozen end. It made a world of difference for them to be able to hold it on their own.

One of the most unexpected tricks I found was with toothbrushes. When I would brush their teeth, they'd keep their mouths open like they were supposed to—until they started teething. Suddenly, they'd try to chew on the toothbrush for relief. So, I went to the store and bought a whole bunch of toothbrushes, giving them as teething toys. They could gnaw on the bristles, and it seemed to hit just the right spots.

I tried everything I could think of for each child, experimenting until I found what worked best. From teething tablets to frozen toys, each one had their favorite way of getting through the pain, and in time, I learned exactly how to help soothe them.

These methods can help ease your baby's discomfort during teething, but every baby responds differently, so it's important to try what works best for your little one.

Chapter 8
Dealing with Rashes

Common Infant and Toddler Rashes

1. Diaper Rash (Irritant Contact Dermatitis)
   - What it looks like: Red, irritated patches in the diaper area.
   - Painful?: Can be mild to moderate discomfort, particularly when touched.
   - How it spreads: Not contagious, caused by wetness, friction, or irritants in diapers.
   - Prevention: Change diapers frequently, use a barrier cream.
   - Treatment: Apply diaper creams containing zinc oxide, make your own with coconut oil and cornstarch, use breast milk, keep the area clean and dry.

2. Eczema (Atopic Dermatitis)
   - What it looks like: Dry, scaly patches, often on the face, elbows, or knees.
   - Painful?: Can be itchy and inflamed.
   - How it spreads: Not contagious, typically a genetic predisposition to sensitive skin.
   - Prevention: Avoid harsh soaps, keep skin moisturized, and manage triggers (e.g., certain fabrics).
   - Treatment: Use emollients, topical corticosteroids for flare-ups, and antihistamines for itching.

3. Hand, Foot, and Mouth Disease
   - What it looks like: Red spots on hands, feet, and mouth (sometimes with blisters).
   - Painful?: Mild fever, sore throat, and mouth ulcers can cause discomfort.
   - How it spreads: Highly contagious through saliva, stool, or respiratory droplets.

   - Prevention: Wash hands frequently, avoid close contact with infected individuals.
   - Treatment: Pain relief with acetaminophen, maintain hydration, and mouth care to soothe ulcers.

4. Teething Rash
   - What it looks like: Red, bumpy rash around the mouth, chin, or sometimes neck, often due to excessive drooling.
   - Painful?: Typically not painful, but can be irritating.
   - How it spreads: Not contagious, associated with increased drooling during teething.
   - Prevention: Use a bib to absorb drool, wipe the face regularly, and keep the area dry.
   - Treatment: Apply a gentle moisturizer, clean the area regularly to prevent skin irritation, and use teething rings for comfort.
   - Additional Note: Teething can also lead to diaper rashes because of increased saliva production, which may irritate the skin in the diaper area, especially when it comes into contact with urine or stool more often due to drooling.

5. Rashes from Repeated Touching or Licking
   - What it looks like: Red, irritated patches where a child repeatedly licks, touches, or rubs a specific area, such as a wrist, cheek, or elbow.
   - Painful?: The rash is usually not painful but can become sore or inflamed if scratched or further irritated.
   - How it spreads: Not contagious, but can worsen if the child continues the behavior.
   - Prevention: Gently discourage the child from licking or rubbing the same spot repeatedly. Use bandages or mittens if necessary.
   - Treatment: Apply a soothing moisturizer to the affected area, and consider using a mild corticosteroid cream for inflammation.

6.Food Sensitivity Rash (Allergic Reaction)
  - What it looks like: Red, raised hives or welts, typically on the face or torso.
  - Painful?: Can be itchy, sometimes with swelling.
  - How it spreads: Triggered by allergens in food (e.g., milk, eggs, peanuts).
  - Prevention: Avoid known allergens, consult an allergist.
  - Treatment: Antihistamines for mild reactions, epinephrine for severe anaphylaxis.

7. Milk Sensitivity Rash
  - What it looks like: Eczema-like rash, especially on cheeks or chin.
  - Painful?: Itchy or mildly painful.
  - How it spreads: Caused by cow's milk proteins in breastmilk or formula.
  - Prevention: Eliminate milk from the diet if sensitivity is suspected.
  - Treatment: Change to hypoallergenic formula or avoid dairy in the breastfeeding mother's diet.

8. Hives (Urticaria)
  - What it looks like: Raised, red, itchy welts that vary in size.
  - Painful?: Can be very itchy.
  - How it spreads: Not contagious, often caused by allergic reactions to food, medications, or environmental factors.
  - Prevention: Avoid known allergens.
  - Treatment: Antihistamines, and in severe cases, steroids.

9. Contact Dermatitis (Allergic or Irritant)
  - What it looks like: Red, inflamed rash in response to an irritant or allergen (e.g., certain soaps, lotions, or plants like poison ivy).
  - Painful?: Can be itchy or burn.
  - How it spreads: Not contagious, caused by contact with allergens or irritants.
  - Prevention: Avoid known triggers.
  - Treatment: Avoid exposure, use antihistamines or topical steroids

10. Heat Rash (Prickly Heat)
   - What it looks like: Small, red bumps, usually in areas that sweat.
   - Painful?: Itchy and may feel prickly.
   - How it spreads: Not contagious, caused by sweat trapped in the sweat
glands.
   - Prevention: Keep the child cool, dress in loose-fitting clothes.
   - Treatment: Cool baths and calamine lotion to soothe itching.

11. Molluscum Contagiosum
   - What it looks like: Small, flesh-colored bumps with a dimple in the
center.
   - Painful?: Not painful, but can become irritated if scratched.
   - How it spreads: Highly contagious, spread by skin-to-skin contact.
   - Prevention: Avoid contact with infected skin, wash hands regularly.
   - Treatment: Typically resolves on its own, but treatments may include
cryotherapy or topical medications.

12.Cradle Cap (Infantile Seborrheic Dermatitis)
- What it looks like: Cradle cap appears as yellow, greasy, scaly patches on
the scalp, sometimes extending to the eyebrows or behind the ears. The
scales can be thick and crusty.
   - Painful?: Cradle cap is generally not painful or itchy, though it may cause
mild irritation in some cases.
- How it spreads: Not contagious. It is caused by an overproduction of oils
in the skin's sebaceous glands, which can be triggered by hormonal
changes from the mother during pregnancy or overactive sebaceous
glands in the baby.
- Prevention: While cradle cap can't always be prevented, keeping the
baby's scalp clean and gently washing it can help. Avoid using harsh
shampoos or scrubbing too hard, as this can irritate the skin.
- Treatment:
   - Use a mild baby shampoo to wash the scalp regularly.
   - After bathing, gently rub the scalp with a soft brush to loosen the flakes.

- Apply natural oils, such as olive oil or coconut oil, to the scalp for 10–15 minutes before washing to soften the scales, making them easier to remove.

- If the condition persists or is severe, consult a pediatrician, who may recommend medicated shampoos or topical treatments.

13. Ringworm (Tinea Corporis)
- What it looks like: Circular red patches with a raised border and clear center.
- Painful?: Typically not painful but can be itchy.
- How it spreads: Contagious, spread by direct contact or contaminated surfaces.
- Prevention: Avoid sharing personal items, wash hands frequently.
- Treatment: Antifungal creams or oral medication.

14. Scabies
- What it looks like: Red, pimple-like rash with small blisters and tunnels under the skin.
- Painful?: Itchy, especially at night.
- How it spreads: Highly contagious, spread by skin-to-skin contact.
- Prevention: Avoid contact with infected individuals.
- Treatment: Prescription creams or oral medications.

15. Rubella (German Measles)
- What it looks like: Pink or red rash that starts on the face and spreads downward.
- Painful?: Mild fever and sore throat, but the rash itself is not painful.
- How it spreads: Highly contagious, spread through respiratory droplets.
- Prevention: Vaccination (MMR).
- Treatment: Supportive care (rest, fluids, and fever reducers).

16. Coxsackievirus Rash
   - What it looks like: Small red spots or bumps, often with white centers, that appear on hands, feet, and buttocks.
   - Painful?: Can be itchy and uncomfortable.
   - How it spreads: Spread through contact with infected saliva or stool.
   - Prevention: Wash hands frequently, avoid contact with infected individuals.
   - Treatment: Pain relief and hydration, rash usually resolves on its own.

17. Lichen Simplex Chronicus
   - What it looks like: Thick, scaly patches of skin that may be darker than surrounding skin.
   - Painful?: Itchy, especially when the skin is scratched.
   - How it spreads: Not contagious, caused by chronic scratching or rubbing.
   - Prevention: Avoid scratching and keep the skin moisturized.
   - Treatment: Topical steroids and antihistamines for itching.

18. Impetigo
   - What it looks like: Blisters that burst, leaving honey-colored crusts.
   - Painful?: Can be itchy and tender.
   - How it spreads: Highly contagious, spread by direct contact with the sores or infected items.
   - Prevention: Wash hands frequently, avoid contact with infected areas.
   - Treatment: Topical or oral antibiotics.

19. Slapped Cheek Syndrome (Parvovirus B19)
   - What it looks like: Red rash on cheeks (like slapped), followed by a lacy rash on limbs.
   - Painful?: Mild fever and malaise, but not painful.
   - How it spreads: Spread through respiratory droplets.
   - Prevention: Wash hands frequently, avoid close contact with infected individuals.

- Treatment: Usually resolves on its own, treat symptoms with fever reducers.

20. Chickenpox (Varicella)
   - What it looks like: Itchy red spots that turn into fluid-filled blisters, then crust over.
   - Painful?: The blisters are very itchy and can be painful.
   - How it spreads: Highly contagious through respiratory droplets or contact with the fluid from the blisters.
   - Prevention: Vaccination and avoiding contact with infected individuals.
   - Treatment: Calamine lotion, antihistamines, and pain relievers to control itching.

When Lilly, my first daughter, was born, we noticed something wasn't quite right. Just a few weeks into breastfeeding, she started developing rashes along with other symptoms like fussiness and digestive issues. At first, I didn't think too much of it, assuming it was just baby skin being sensitive. But as the rashes persisted, we decided to call the doctor. I was told it might be a skin irritation, but it didn't quite make sense. We kept going to the doctor and treating the rashes with creams and ointments, but nothing seemed to help long-term.

I did some research and began eliminating different foods and lactose from my diet, suspecting that something in my breast milk was causing the reaction. Still, nothing seemed to work. By the time Lilly was a month old, I was exhausted from trying everything, but when we switched to a sensitive formula, everything changed. The rashes cleared up significantly, and she seemed so much more comfortable. It was such a relief to see her finally calm down.

But teething always brought its own set of challenges. With every new tooth, all my babies would get diaper rashes, drool excessively, and have the nastiest, most painful-looking poops. It was like a signal that teething was on its way. I became a pro at using diaper creams and changing them often to avoid any further irritation. I even started making my own diaper cream, mixing coconut oil with cornstarch and alcohol free witch hazel. Coconut oil has anti-inflammatory and moisturizing properties that help soothe irritated skin, while cornstarch absorbs excess moisture and keeps the skin dry. It worked wonders.

Then, there was my stepson, who went to daycare and had his own health battles. He caught hand, foot, and mouth disease multiple times, each time from the daycare. I remember the first time it happened—we were really worried. He was uncomfortable, cuddling up to me and drinking applesauce from a straw. It was hard to watch him suffer, but after the daycare sent out a notice about the outbreak, we realized what it was. It was a big relief to understand the cause of his symptoms.

Daycare felt like a breeding ground for illness, and after dealing with it several times, I decided homeschooling would be a better fit for my other kids. With daycare, we had no control over his attendance, and it just seemed like a constant cycle of sickness. My stepson also had this habit of brushing his cheek with his hand, which eventually led to a rash on his face. He also developed bumps on his arms—little edemas. They didn't seem to bother him, but it was another worry we had to keep an eye on. Looking back, it was a lot to juggle, but each experience taught me something new about how to care for my children's sensitive skin and health.

Looking back, it's clear that every child brought their own set of challenges. With Lilly, it was the food sensitivities and rashes; with my other children, it was teething and diaper rashes, and with my stepson, it was the constant battle with daycare illnesses. But through it all, the more I talked with other moms, consulted with doctors, and did my own research, the better I felt. Each challenge felt a little less daunting when I had the support and knowledge to handle it. With each new child, I felt more prepared, knowing that I had already been through these struggles before. The experiences made me a more confident mom, and I learned that, though every child is different, the ability to adapt and learn as you go can make the journey easier and more manageable.

Remedies that worked

These remedies offer a combination of soothing, anti-inflammatory, and healing properties that can be helpful in treating a variety of rashes in infants and toddlers. Always ensure that any essential oils or products used are properly diluted, and consult your pediatrician before using any new treatment, especially for infants.

1. Coconut Oil and Cornstarch
   - Benefits: Coconut oil has antibacterial, antifungal, and anti-inflammatory properties; cornstarch absorbs moisture.
   - Used for: Diaper rash, skin irritation, and friction-related rashes.
   - How to Use: Mix a small amount of coconut oil with cornstarch and apply to affected areas after bathing.

2. Breastmilk
   - Benefits: Contains antibodies, enzymes, and nutrients that can help soothe and heal skin.
   - Used for: Eczema, diaper rash, and minor skin irritations.
   - How to Use: Apply a small amount directly to the rash and let it air dry.

3. Non-Alcoholic Witch Hazel and Frankincense
   - Benefits: Witch hazel soothes irritation and inflammation; frankincense has anti-inflammatory and healing properties.
   - Used for: Redness, irritation, and minor cuts.
   - How to Use: Mix a few drops of frankincense with witch hazel, then apply using a cotton ball or as a wipe.

4. Aloe Vera Gel
   - Benefits: Hydrates, reduces inflammation, and speeds healing.
   - Used for: Mild sunburn, skin irritation, and eczema.
   - How to Use: Apply a thin layer of pure aloe vera gel to the affected area.

5. Oatmeal Bath (Colloidal Oatmeal)
   - Benefits: Soothes itching, calms inflammation, and moisturizes skin.
   - Used for: Eczema, chickenpox, and dry skin.
   - How to Use: Add colloidal oatmeal to a warm bath and let your child soak for 10–15 minutes.

6. Coconut Oil
   - Benefits: Moisturizes skin, reduces redness, and has antifungal and antibacterial properties.
   - Used for: Diaper rash, eczema, and dry skin.
   - How to Use: Apply directly to the affected area after bathing.

7. Calendula Cream
   - Benefits: Reduces inflammation and promotes skin healing.
   - Used for: Diaper rash, cuts, and mild skin irritations.
   - How to Use: Apply a thin layer of calendula cream to the rash.

8. Zinc Oxide Cream
   - Benefits: Forms a barrier to protect the skin and reduces irritation.
   - Used for: Diaper rash.
   - How to Use: Apply generously to the diaper area after each diaper change.

9. Hydrocortisone Cream (1%)
   - Benefits: Reduces inflammation and itching.
   - Used for: Eczema, contact dermatitis, and rashes caused by allergic reactions.
   - How to Use: Apply a thin layer to the affected area, but avoid overuse (consult a doctor first).

10. Apple Cider Vinegar
   - Benefits: Has antifungal and antibacterial properties.
   - Used for: Diaper rash and fungal infections.
   - How to Use: Dilute apple cider vinegar with water and apply gently with a cotton ball.

11. Breastmilk Soap
  - Benefits: Breast Milk contains natural fats, vitamins, and antibodies that can help soothe and hydrate irritated skin while promoting healing.
  - Used for: Eczema, diaper rash, dry skin, and minor rashes.
  - How to Use: Use breastmilk soap during bath time to cleanse the skin gently without stripping its natural oils. You can find or make breastmilk soap by incorporating expressed breast milk into a soap base.

12. Lavender Oil
  - Benefits: Calms skin and has soothing anti-inflammatory properties.
  - Used for: Eczema, diaper rash, and general skin irritation.
  - How to Use: Dilute lavender oil with a carrier oil (such as coconut oil) and apply to the rash.

13. Chamomile Tea Compress
  - Benefits: Soothes and calms irritated skin.
  - Used for: Eczema, rashes, and skin irritation.
  - How to Use: Brew chamomile tea, let it cool, then use a cloth to apply it as a compress.

14. Epsom Salt Bath
  - Benefits: Relieves itching and calms inflammation.
  - Used for: Eczema, insect bites, and general skin irritation.
  - How to Use: Add a small amount of Epsom salt to a warm bath and allow your child to soak for 15–20 minutes.

15. Tea Tree Oil (Diluted)
  - Benefits: Antiseptic and antifungal properties.
  - Used for: Fungal rashes, diaper rash, and eczema.
  - How to Use: Dilute tea tree oil with a carrier oil and apply to the affected area.

16. Cucumber Slices
  - Benefits: Cooling and moisturizing.
  - Used for: Heat rash and irritated skin.
  - How to Use: Place fresh cucumber slices on the rash or gently rub the juice from the cucumber on the affected area.

17. Lemon Balm
  - Benefits: Soothes itching and reduces inflammation.
  - Used for: Chickenpox, insect bites, and minor rashes.
  - How to Use: Apply lemon balm cream or tea to the affected area.

18. Petroleum Jelly (Vaseline)
  - Benefits: Creates a barrier that helps lock in moisture and protect from further irritation.
  - Used for: Diaper rash, dry skin, and cracked skin.
  - How to Use: Apply to the affected area after a bath to seal in moisture.

19. Breast Milk for Eczema or Diaper Rash
  - Benefits: Contains natural antibodies and helps soothe irritation.
  - Used for: Eczema, minor rashes, and diaper rash.
  - How to Use: Express a small amount of breast milk and apply directly to the rash.

20. Non-Alcoholic Witch Hazel
  - Benefits: Reduces inflammation, soothes irritation, and tightens skin.
  - Used for: Minor skin irritations, cuts, and rashes.
  - How to Use: Apply witch hazel to a cotton ball and gently dab it on the affected skin.

When my kids were babies, their skin was incredibly sensitive. It seemed like no matter what I tried, there was always a rash lurking around the corner. Some creams and ointments I used helped a little, but they often caused new problems. The harsh chemicals, though effective in reducing the rash, irritated their delicate skin even more, leaving me feeling helpless. It was a constant cycle of trying new things, only to see them struggle with something else.

I remember countless nights staring at the medicine cabinet, wondering what would work without causing more issues. I felt like I was running out of options until I decided to dive in deep—researching, asking other moms, and consulting with doctors. I was determined to find a solution that wouldn't just mask the problem but would actually help heal their sensitive skin.

It wasn't long before I began exploring natural remedies. I started experimenting with things like coconut oil, which is known for its anti-inflammatory properties, and natural butters, which are gentle on skin and keep it moisturized. Breast milk, too, proved to be a surprising ally—it helped soothe rashes and irritation in a way that commercial creams never could. I even came across things like chamomile and aloe vera, which had a calming effect and made a noticeable difference.

Slowly but surely, I began to notice a change. My kids' rashes became less frequent, and when they did appear, they were much less severe. I had found a routine that worked for them, and it didn't involve any harsh chemicals. The more I used these natural remedies, the more confident I became in my ability to manage their sensitive skin. I even started using some of these solutions on myself and my husband, and to my surprise, they worked just as well for us.

Now, it's very rare for my kids to get a rash. When they do, I know exactly what to do, and I don't panic like I used to. What once seemed like an endless cycle of irritation and frustration has turned into a manageable part of life. Looking back, I'm grateful for the journey I took to figure out what worked for my kids' skin. I learned a lot about what their bodies needed, and now, we all benefit from the simple, effective remedies that have become a part of our daily routine. It's one of those things that makes me feel like a bit of a skin care expert for my own home, and I'm so glad I stuck with it, even when things felt uncertain.

What to watch for and when to call the doctor

1. Redness and Inflammation – If the rash spreads quickly or becomes red and swollen, it might be a sign of infection.

2. Fever with Rash – A fever accompanying the rash could indicate a viral or bacterial infection. Call the doctor if the fever is 100.4°F (38°C) or higher.

3. Pus or Blisters – If the rash starts to ooze pus or blisters form, it could indicate a bacterial infection, like impetigo.

4. Rashes that don't fade – Pressing on the rash and seeing if it fades (blanching) is key. If it doesn't, this could be a sign of something serious, like meningitis.

5. Rash with Breathing Difficulty – Seek immediate medical help if the rash is accompanied by trouble breathing or swelling in the lips, tongue, or throat.

6. Peeling Skin – If the rash causes peeling or skin sloughing, it could be a sign of a more serious condition like a drug reaction.

7. Purple Spots or Bruises – Unexplained purple spots or bruises under the skin, known as purpura, require urgent attention as they could indicate bleeding disorders.

8. Itchiness – Mild itchiness can be normal, but extreme itchiness might indicate an allergic reaction or conditions like eczema or hives.

9. Rash on the Face – If the rash is concentrated around the eyes, mouth, or other sensitive areas, monitor closely and consult the doctor if it worsens.

10. Spread to Other Parts – If a rash spreads to other parts of the body quickly, it might need medical evaluation to rule out an infection or allergic reaction.

11. Rash Caused by New Foods – A rash following the introduction of new foods could indicate a food allergy. Watch for other symptoms, like swelling or vomiting, and contact the doctor.

12. Rash Lasting More Than a Few Days – If the rash doesn't clear up in a few days, call the doctor to see if treatment is needed.

13. Severe Diaper Rash – If diaper rash is severe, not improving with over-the-counter creams, or has open sores, it may require medical attention.

14. Dry, Scaly, or Cracked Skin – Persistent dryness, especially if it cracks, could be eczema or dermatitis and may require prescription creams or other treatments.

15. Rash After Vaccinations – Some vaccinations may cause mild rashes, but if the rash is severe or accompanied by other symptoms, contact your doctor.

16. Rash After Medication – A rash after starting a new medication could be a drug reaction, especially if there are other symptoms like swelling, difficulty breathing, or a widespread rash.

17. Rash Around the Mouth or Chin – This could be a drool rash. If it becomes red, inflamed, or doesn't improve with basic care, check with the doctor.

18. Hand, Foot, and Mouth Disease Symptoms – Watch for red spots, ulcers, or a rash on the palms, soles, and inside the mouth. Contact the doctor for advice on symptom management.

19. Swollen Lymph Nodes – If a rash is accompanied by swollen lymph nodes, it may be due to an infection that requires medical evaluation.

20. Persistent or Recurrent Rashes – If a rash keeps returning or doesn't go away after typical home care, it could indicate a chronic condition like eczema, psoriasis, or a fungal infection, requiring a doctor's assessment.

When my stepson and first daughter were little, I felt like I was always calling the doctor. Every small rash or symptom would send me into a state of worry, and by the time we got to the doctor's office, I'd have a long list of questions ready. I'd watch the doctor's face as I went through them, half-expecting them to tell me I was overreacting. But usually, my instincts were correct.

The trouble was, I was new to being a parent, and I didn't trust myself. Every small hiccup in their health felt like a potential crisis, and I needed reassurance that I was doing the right thing. I didn't realize back then that it was okay not to have all the answers, that I would learn in time. As a new mom, the idea of "overprotective" hung over me like a cloud, but I'd rather be that than regret not doing enough.

As I had more children, I got better. With each new baby, I learned from my past experiences. Things became less scary because I had seen it all before—or so I thought. Then, inevitably, something new would pop up. But by that time, I had learned to trust myself. I wasn't afraid to ask for help, but I also knew when to follow my gut and just take a breath.

I've realized that being a mother means learning constantly, trusting your instincts, and knowing that sometimes it's okay to ask for help. I'd rather be overprotective than a sorry mother. And when it comes to things like rashes and illnesses, those guidelines can help with monitoring, but always trust your instincts and call the doctor if you're unsure. After all, that's how we grow as parents—by caring deeply, learning from each experience, and never being afraid to ask for guidance when needed.

Chapter 9
Potty Training

Timing Potty Training

1. Look for Readiness Signs
Watch for cues like staying dry for longer periods, showing interest in the toilet, or expressing discomfort with dirty diapers.
-Why: Starting too early can lead to frustration. Waiting until your child is ready makes the process smoother.

2. Introduce the Concept Early
Talk about potty training before starting, read books about it, or let your child observe others using the toilet.
-Why: Familiarizing your child with the idea early helps reduce anxiety and build confidence.

3. Choose the Right Time
Avoid starting during big changes like a new sibling, moving, or daycare transitions.
-Why: Potty training requires focus. Major life changes can create stress and delays in progress.

4. Pick a Potty
Choose a potty chair or seat insert that is comfortable and easy for your child to use.
-Why: Having their own potty creates ownership and reduces fear of the big toilet.

5. Set a Routine
Start with regular potty trips, like after meals or waking up, and build them into your daily schedule.
-Why: Consistency helps your child recognize when it's time to go, establishing a pattern.

6. Use Positive Reinforcement
Offer praise, stickers, or small rewards when your child uses the potty
successfully.
-Why: Positive reinforcement encourages repeat behavior and builds your
child's confidence.

7. Dress for Success
Use easy-to-remove clothes like elastic waistbands or training pants.
-Why: Clothes that are tricky to remove can cause accidents and
frustration.

8. Make Potty Time Fun
Bring toys, books, or sing songs while they sit on the potty.
-Why: Keeping the experience fun and relaxed helps reduce any pressure
or fear.

9. Introduce Underwear as a Milestone
Let your child pick out special "big kid" underwear once they've made
progress.
-Why: Wearing underwear feels like an achievement and motivates them to
stay dry.

10. Start with Daytime Training
Focus on getting them dry during the day before tackling naps or nighttime
training.
-Why: Daytime training is usually easier, and once mastered, your child will
be more ready for the next step.

11. Be Patient with Accidents
Respond calmly to accidents by reassuring your child and helping them
clean up.
-Why: Frustration can cause setbacks. Keeping calm reinforces that
accidents are part of learning.

12. Encourage Independence
Let your child pull down their pants, sit on the potty, and wipe themselves (with supervision).
-Why: Fostering independence builds confidence and helps them feel in control of the process.

13. Teach Hygiene Early
Show them how to wipe properly, wash hands after using the toilet, and use flushable wipes if needed.
-Why: Establishing good hygiene habits early prevents health issues and reinforces the complete process.

14. Stay Consistent Across Environments
Ensure the same potty training rules apply at home, daycare, or with other caregivers.
-Why: Consistency helps avoid confusion and keeps the training process moving forward smoothly.

15. Use a Timer or Reminder
Set a timer for regular potty breaks or remind your child every hour or two.
-Why: Timed reminders help them remember to go before it's too late and establish a habit.

16. Switch to Pull-Ups for Transitioning
Use pull-ups during outings or naps to prevent accidents, but encourage underwear use at home.
-Why: Pull-ups provide a safety net but still allow for easier bathroom access compared to diapers.

17. Celebrate Small Wins
Celebrate every small success, like going to the potty or staying dry for an hour.
-Why: Acknowledging progress keeps your child motivated and excited about learning.

18. Track Progress
Keep a chart of successes, accidents, and patterns to see where your child
is improving.
-Why: Tracking helps you see what's working, and where your child might
need extra encouragement.

19. Introduce Night Training Gradually
Once your child is consistently dry during the day, try limiting fluids before
bedtime and using nighttime pull-ups as a transition.
-Why: Night training takes longer, and doing it gradually can prevent
unnecessary frustration.

20. Stay Calm and Flexible
If your child shows resistance or isn't progressing, take a break and try
again later.
-Why: Pushing too hard can lead to power struggles or setbacks. A flexible
approach helps maintain a positive experience for both you and your child.

When I potty trained my first two and last toddler, it felt like a breeze. They were all fully trained by the time they turned two. After my first two I didn't quite understand why people said, "Wait until they're ready." I thought I had it all figured out. But then came my third child, and she threw every plan out the window. I was determined to get her trained by two as well, but she had other ideas. She wouldn't even sit on the toilet, and no amount of coaxing or encouragement seemed to work.

The experience was humbling. I had to put aside my expectations and go all the way back to the basics. Instead of pushing, I started taking her to the bathroom with me, hoping she'd catch on by watching. And sure enough, when she was ready, everything started to click. It became clear she needed to go at her own pace. Things went much smoother after that, and she made it just before her second birthday, but not without a struggle.

My other kids were easier in comparison. The hardest part for me wasn't getting them to go—it was committing to the life of always having to make the first stop the potty. Spending so much time in the bathroom became our new normal. But my kids loved the routines, and the charts made it fun for them. Eventually, they started going to the bathroom without me. It was one of those bittersweet moments—on one hand, I was relieved they could do it on their own, but on the other, it was a little sad to watch them grow so independent.

Training Tips for Busy Parents

1. Create a Potty Training Schedule
Set regular potty times (e.g., after meals, before naps, before leaving the house).
-Why: A routine helps children recognize when it's time to go, building a habit that reduces accidents.

2. Have Siblings Go Together
Bring two or more kids to the bathroom at the same time, if possible.
-Why: It saves time and helps younger children learn by watching their siblings, encouraging a team effort.

3. Use a Potty Training Chart
Create a reward chart where each child earns a sticker or mark for every successful potty trip.
-Why: Visual progress motivates kids and gives them a sense of achievement.

4. Utilize Bathroom Time for Yourself
Keep a small set of hand weights in the bathroom for quick workouts, or bring a book to read while supervising.
-Why: It turns what can feel like wasted time into productive "me-time" for physical or mental well-being.

5. Pack Portable Potty Seats
Keep portable potty seats in the car or diaper bag.
-Why: Being prepared during outings prevents accidents and encourages consistency when away from home.

6. Stick to the Routine Even if They Don't Go
Bring your child to the bathroom at regular intervals, even if they don't use the potty.
-Why: Consistency is key to building the habit of sitting on the potty, and eventually, they'll start using it regularly.

7. Set a Timer for Regular Potty Breaks
Use a timer to remind yourself and your kids to visit the potty every 30–60 minutes.
-Why: A timer helps you stay consistent even during busy days, and kids start recognizing when it's time to go.

8. Keep Extra Clothes Handy
Have an easily accessible bag of extra clothes, underwear, and wipes in case of accidents.
-Why: Being prepared for accidents keeps the stress level low and avoids unnecessary delays in your day.

9. Encourage Independent Dressing
Teach your child to pull down their pants and underwear by themselves.
-Why: Encouraging independence reduces the need for you to help each time and speeds up the process.

10. Praise Effort, Not Just Success
Give praise for trying, even if they don't succeed in going potty.
-Why: Positive reinforcement encourages effort and reduces anxiety or fear of failure.

11. Use Rewards Sparingly
Offer small rewards like stickers or a special activity for potty success, but don't overdo it.
-Why: Too many rewards can lead to dependency, but small incentives motivate without overwhelming.

12. Teach Hygiene Early
Show your kids how to wipe properly, wash hands, and flush after using the potty.
-Why: Establishing these habits early prevents hygiene issues and encourages independence.

13. Make Potty Time Fun
Let your kids bring a favorite book or toy into the bathroom or play fun
songs while they sit.
-Why: Keeping it fun helps reduce stress, making them more willing to sit
on the potty.

14. Stay Calm During Accidents
Respond calmly to accidents, remind your child to try again next time, and
clean up together.
-Why: Staying calm reassures your child and keeps the potty training
process positive.

15. Use Pull-Ups for Night and Outings
Use pull-ups at night or during long outings, but encourage underwear
during the day.
-Why: Pull-ups provide a safety net without undoing progress, giving your
child confidence while avoiding accidents.

16. Set Up a Potty Station
Create a bathroom station with everything your child needs—wipes, extra
clothes, and a potty chart—so it's always ready.
-Why: A prepared station reduces time spent running around and keeps the
routine consistent.

17. Turn It Into a Game
Make up a potty song, race to the potty, or use fun phrases when it's time
to go.
-Why: Turning potty time into a playful game keeps kids engaged and
excited.

18. Make the Potty Accessible
Use potty chairs or stools so kids can easily get on and off the toilet by
themselves.
-Why: Easy access fosters independence and builds confidence in using
the potty on their own.

19. Limit Drinks Before Bedtime
Gradually reduce liquids an hour before bed to help with nighttime potty training.
-Why: This reduces the likelihood of accidents during the night and helps establish dry nights.

20. Be Flexible and Don't Rush
If your child isn't ready, take a break and try again in a few weeks.
-Why: Rushing or forcing potty training can cause resistance. Flexibility ensures the process happens when your child is truly ready.

In our house, potty time was never just another task—it was a celebration! We made it a fun, lively event right from the start. Every trip to the potty turned into a little party, complete with songs and dances. We'd sing a silly potty song on the way to the bathroom, and when they finished, it was like they just won a prize. The kids loved it, and it made the whole process feel like an exciting adventure instead of something stressful.

At the beginning, potty time was the highlight of the day. We'd all get so excited, clapping and cheering when they sat on the potty, even if they didn't actually go. As they got older, the fun didn't stop. The older ones started imitating me, guiding their younger siblings to the potty just like I had done with them. It turned into a playful family activity, with the older ones becoming little "potty coaches," which made them feel important and kept the fun alive.

We had a rewards system in stages, which kept the motivation going. First, they'd get a sticker or a small treat just for sitting on the potty, even if nothing happened. Then, the rewards shifted to when they actually went potty, and finally, for going poop. But sometimes, they didn't get a reward when they were expecting one, and that was hard—for both of us. There were moments when I wanted to give in and hand over a treat just to avoid the disappointment in their eyes, but I knew I had to stay strong. Instead, I'd say, "Good job trying! Maybe next time, we'll get that reward."

Eventually, something amazing happened. They no longer needed the rewards to go. They just started doing it all on their own, without needing any prompting. It was bittersweet. I was so proud of them for being independent, but at the same time, it meant my role in the potty party was slowly fading. But that's how it goes—they grow, they learn, and before you know it, they're off handling things like little pros.

Handling Setbacks

1. Stay Patient
Take deep breaths and remind yourself that setbacks are normal. Avoid showing frustration in front of your child.
-Why: Children pick up on stress, and staying calm will help them feel secure and more willing to keep trying.

2. Offer Gentle Encouragement
Reassure your child that it's okay if they have an accident. Use phrases like, "You'll get it next time!"
-Why: Positive reinforcement helps them feel confident, and less stressed about mistakes.

3. Revisit the Basics
If your child is struggling, go back to simple potty steps, like sitting on the potty fully clothed.
-Why: It breaks down the process and helps rebuild their confidence.

4. Use a Timer Again
If your child is having frequent accidents, set a timer to remind both of you to try using the potty every 30-45 minutes.
-Why: Frequent reminders help re-establish the routine and prevent accidents.

5. Keep Extra Clothes Handy
Always have a bag with extra underwear, clothes, and wipes in case of accidents, whether at home or on the go.
-Why: Being prepared reduces stress when accidents happen and helps keep the day moving smoothly.

6. Avoid Punishment
If your child has an accident, simply clean up and remind them that it's part of learning.
-Why: Punishment can make children anxious or resistant, while patience encourages progress.

7. Offer More Rewards for Effort
Give praise or small rewards like stickers even if they don't successfully go potty but try.
-Why: Reinforcing effort helps them feel accomplished and motivated to keep going.

8. Use Visual Reminders
Post a chart or picture in the bathroom to remind them of each step (e.g., pull down pants, sit, go, wipe, flush, wash hands).
-Why: Visual cues are helpful for younger children who may forget what to do next.

9. Monitor Liquid Intake
Be mindful of how much your child drinks, especially close to naptime or bedtime.
-Why: Less liquid before naps and nighttime reduces the chance of accidents, which can help avoid setbacks.

10. Reinforce a Potty Routine
Stick to a regular schedule for potty breaks even if your child doesn't feel the urge to go.
-Why: A structured routine reinforces the habit and can help prevent accidents over time.

11. Stay Consistent, Even During Setbacks
Stick with your potty training routine and avoid taking long breaks unless absolutely necessary.
-Why: Consistency helps your child understand the expectations and reduces confusion.

12. Focus on Hygiene After Accidents

Use accidents as teaching moments for hygiene, having your child help clean up and wash their hands afterward.

-Why: Teaching hygiene in this context helps them understand it's part of the process without making accidents a big deal.

13. Incorporate Potty Time into Play

Use a doll or stuffed animal to role-play potty time.

-Why: Playing out the scenario with toys makes it fun and helps your child feel more comfortable with the process.

14. Give Them Control Over Underwear Choice

Let your child pick out special "big kid" underwear with characters or colors they like.

-Why: Giving them a sense of ownership motivates them to keep their underwear dry.

15. Try Different Potty Options

If your child is resisting, experiment with a different potty chair or a seat on the regular toilet.

-Why: Sometimes a change in equipment helps them feel more comfortable or curious about trying again.

16. Don't Rush Out of Pull-Ups Too Soon

If accidents are frequent, use pull-ups for outings or during naps and nights until they're more consistent.

-Why: It helps avoid messes while allowing your child to continue practicing without feeling pressured.

17. Be Mindful of Distractions

Limit distractions (like screen time) close to potty times to encourage focus.

-Why: Kids can easily get too distracted to remember to go potty, leading to accidents.

18. Encourage Potty Breaks Before Transitions
Have your child use the potty before meals, outings, or naps.
-Why: Reinforcing potty breaks during key transition times helps prevent
accidents and maintains the habit.

19. Celebrate Small Wins
Celebrate every milestone, whether it's sitting on the potty, pulling down
pants independently, or using the potty once during a rough day.
-Why: Recognizing small steps keeps the experience positive and helps
them stay motivated during setbacks.

20. Seek Support if Needed
If progress stalls or you feel overwhelmed, talk to your pediatrician or other
parents for advice and reassurance.
-Why: Sometimes setbacks are a normal part of the process, but getting
expert advice can help ease concerns and identify solutions.

These tips are designed to help handle setbacks with patience,
persistence, and creativity, keeping the process low-stress for both you and
your kids while staying on track.

Potty training in our house wasn't just about learning when and how to go—it was about sticking to a routine that kept us on track. For us, routines and sometimes even a timer were key. Every couple of min- couple of hours, I'd remind them it was time to sit on the potty, even if they didn't think they had to go. We made it a regular part of the day, whether we were playing, eating, or getting ready for bed. It worked because the kids knew what to expect, and I could count on fewer accidents.

But, of course, life doesn't always stick to a routine. If we had visitors, or when we went on vacation, things would shift. We'd get off schedule, and I'd notice little regressions here and there. It was frustrating, especially when we had been doing so well, but I reminded myself that it was okay. Setbacks happen. I knew that we'd get back on track eventually, so I kept trying and didn't let those moments throw us off completely.

One thing that was really important to me was making sure the kids didn't feel embarrassed when accidents happened. After all, they're called accidents for a reason—they can't help it! Instead of reacting negatively, I'd simply say, "Uh oh, let's get cleaned up." We'd clean up together, and then I'd have them sit on the potty, even if they had already gone. They usually didn't have to go again, but sitting on the potty afterward gave us a chance to talk about it. I'd gently remind them, "Next time, we're going to try and go on the potty, so we can get a treat!"

This approach seemed to work because it kept the whole process positive. It helped them understand what went wrong without making them feel bad about it. They were excited for next time, knowing they had another chance to get it right. More than anything, it helped keep their confidence high, and I think that's part of the reason why they kept progressing, even after a rough day.

Chapter 10
Meal Planning for a Busy Household

Simple and Nutritious Meals for the Whole Family

1. One-Pot Meals
Cook everything in a single pot—start with a protein (like chicken or beans),
then add veggies, grains (like quinoa or rice), and liquid (broth or water).
Simmer until everything is tender.
-Benefit: Saves time on prep and cleanup while providing a balanced meal.

2. Sheet Pan Dinners
Arrange proteins (like chicken breasts or tofu) and vegetables on a baking
sheet. Drizzle with olive oil and season, then roast in the oven at 400°F for
25-30 minutes.
-Benefit: Everything cooks together, minimizing cleanup and ensuring even
cooking.

3. Batch Cooking
Double or triple recipes for things like soups, casseroles, or grains, and
freeze or refrigerate leftovers for future meals.
-Benefit: Reduces daily cooking and ensures you always have healthy
meals ready to go.

4. Smoothie Bowls
Blend frozen fruits, greens, yogurt, and milk until smooth. Pour into a bowl
and top with nuts, seeds, and granola for added texture and nutrients.
-Benefit: Packed with vitamins and protein, easy to customize, and great for
sneaking in extra veggies.

5. Breakfast for Dinner
Make scrambled eggs, whole wheat toast, and sautéed veggies for a
simple dinner. Serve with fruit on the side for a balanced meal.
-Benefit: Quick to make, fun for kids, and nutritious with protein, fiber, and
healthy fats.

6. Slow Cooker/Instant Pot Meals
Place your ingredients (meat, veggies, broth) in a slow cooker or Instant
Pot. Set to cook for 4-8 hours (slow cooker) or 15-30 minutes (Instant Pot)
depending on the recipe.
-Benefit: Minimal effort for cooking, allowing you to "set it and forget it"
while preparing nutritious meals.

7. Make-Your-Own Wraps
Lay out whole wheat wraps, lean proteins (chicken, turkey), veggies
(lettuce, tomatoes, peppers), and healthy spreads (hummus, avocado). Let
everyone assemble their own.
-Benefit: Encourages individual preferences while keeping it healthy and
fun for the whole family.

8. Pre-Chopped Veggies
Pre-chop vegetables like carrots, peppers, and cucumbers at the beginning
of the week and store them in airtight containers. Use them for quick
snacks or to throw into meals.
-Benefit: Saves time and makes it easy to add veggies to every meal.

9. Frozen Veggies and Fruits
Keep bags of frozen veggies and fruits in the freezer. Add frozen
vegetables to stir-fries, soups, or casseroles, and use frozen fruits in
smoothies or for snacks.
-Benefit: Just as nutritious as fresh and ready to use at any time, making
meal prep faster.

10. Muffin Tin Meals
Use muffin tins to make mini frittatas, meatloaf, or muffin-shaped meals. Fill
each cup with protein, veggies, and grains, then bake until firm.
-Benefit: Perfect for portion control and fun for kids to eat.

11. Healthy Stir-Fries
Sauté protein (chicken, tofu) in a large pan, then add chopped vegetables.
Stir in a simple sauce made from soy sauce, garlic, and ginger. Serve over
brown rice or noodles.
-Benefit: Fast to make and full of fiber, protein, and essential nutrients.

12. Pasta with Veggie-Packed Sauces
Purée steamed vegetables (like carrots, spinach, or zucchini) into your
favorite pasta sauce. Toss with whole grain pasta and top with a sprinkle of
cheese.
-Benefit: Adds extra vegetables to a family-favorite meal without
compromising flavor.

13. Homemade Pizzas
Use whole wheat pizza dough or flatbreads. Top with tomato sauce,
veggies, and lean proteins (chicken, turkey pepperoni), and bake until
crispy.
-Benefit: Healthier than takeout and lets the family customize toppings to
their liking.

14. Soup and Sandwich Night
Make a simple vegetable or chicken soup and pair it with whole grain
sandwiches filled with lean proteins and veggies.
-Benefit: Easy to prepare, customizable, and a good balance of protein,
carbs, and vegetables.

15. DIY Salad Bar
Set out a variety of greens, chopped veggies, proteins (chicken, beans), and healthy toppings (nuts, seeds, avocado) and let everyone build their own salads.
-Benefit: Encourages veggie consumption and allows for individual preferences.

16. Make-Ahead Overnight Oats
Mix oats, milk, yogurt, and fruit in a jar or bowl. Let it sit in the fridge overnight. In the morning, it's ready to eat.
-Benefit: A quick, healthy breakfast that's rich in fiber and protein.

17. Incorporate Beans and Lentils
Add beans or lentils to soups, salads, tacos, or casseroles. Cook them in bulk and freeze for later use.
-Benefit: These are inexpensive, packed with protein and fiber, and keep you full longer.

18. Grain Bowls
Start with a base of quinoa or brown rice. Add roasted veggies, lean protein, and a drizzle of sauce (like tahini or lemon).
-Benefit: Versatile, nutrient-dense, and easy to assemble for everyone's taste.

19. Veggie-Packed Omelets
Whisk eggs, pour into a hot pan, and add chopped veggies, cheese, and proteins. Cook until firm and serve with whole-grain toast.
-Benefit: A quick, balanced meal full of protein and veggies.

20. Homemade Energy Bites
Mix oats, nut butter, honey, and add-ins like flaxseed, chia seeds, or dried fruit. Roll into balls and store in the fridge for quick snacks.
-Benefit: Nutritious, portable snacks full of healthy fats and fiber.
These methods not only simplify meal prep but also keep the whole family eating healthy and balanced meals without extra effort.

Eating together has always been a priority for me, especially with a busy household full of young kids. I think it's so important for us to gather around together, not just for the food, but for the bonding that happens during family meals. Research shows that eating together improves communication, promotes healthier eating habits, and even boosts children's academic success. I've noticed that when we sit down as a family, it gives us a chance to talk, reconnect, and create a routine that my kids look forward to. It's not just about the meal itself—it's about the time spent together.

One of my favorite go-to tools, especially on busy or stressful days, is the crockpot. I love how I can throw everything in early in the day and not have to worry about cooking later when things tend to get hectic. The best part is that I can still make healthy meals for my family even when I don't have much time. I like sneaking vegetables into dishes—like blending spinach into sauces or adding pureed carrots to soups. It's a little trick to make sure my kids are getting the nutrients they need without them even realizing it.

In the end, feeding my kids healthy food and making family mealtime a priority is something I value deeply. Even with the occasional challenges of picky eaters or busy days, I find that these moments together are worth every bit of effort.

Feeding Toddlers and a Newborn at the Same Time

1. Create a Feeding Station for Both
Set up a designated area with everything you need for feeding both the
newborn and toddler (bottles, snacks, water, bibs, etc.).
-Benefit: Helps you stay organized, minimizes interruptions, and keeps
everything within reach.

2. Use a Baby Carrier While Feeding the Toddler
Wear your newborn in a baby carrier or wrap while feeding the toddler in a
high chair or at the table.
-Benefit: Keeps the newborn close and content while freeing your hands to
focus on feeding the toddler.

3. Feed the Newborn First
Breastfeed or bottle-feed the newborn before sitting down to feed the
toddler. This ensures the baby is full and calm while you focus on the
toddler's meal.
-Benefit: Reduces crying or fussing from the newborn, allowing for a more
peaceful mealtime with the toddler.

4. Offer the Toddler a Snack During Newborn's Feeding Time
Provide a small, healthy snack to the toddler (like fruit, crackers, or cheese)
while you're feeding the newborn.
-Benefit: Keeps the toddler busy and prevents them from getting cranky
while you're occupied.

5. Meal Prep in Advance
Prepare meals or snacks ahead of time for both the toddler and newborn
(pre-chop veggies, prep bottles, etc.).
-Benefit: Saves time and stress when feeding both children, especially
during busy moments.

6. Use Toddler-Friendly Feeding Tools
Give the toddler self-feeding tools like a divided plate, easy-to-grip utensils,
or a sippy cup.
-Benefit: Encourages independence, making it easier for you to focus on
the newborn while the toddler feeds themselves.

7. Offer Simple, Nutritious Finger Foods for the Toddler
Provide the toddler with easy-to-eat finger foods like diced fruit, cheese
cubes, or veggies while feeding the newborn.
-Benefit: Minimizes mess and encourages self-feeding, freeing you up to
care for the baby.

8. Tandem Feed in the Same Room
Feed the toddler and newborn in the same space—sit the toddler at the
table while you bottle-feed or breastfeed the newborn.
-Benefit: Keeps both children close, making it easier to monitor them and
ensuring you can tend to both if needed.

9. Use a Booster Seat or High Chair for the Toddler
Place the toddler in a high chair or booster seat during meal times to keep
them seated and focused on eating.
-Benefit: Contains the toddler in one place, making it easier to manage both
children during feeding times.

10. Synchronize Feeding Schedules
Align the toddler's meal and the newborn's feeding time as closely as possible, so both children are eating at the same time.
-Benefit: Streamlines the feeding process, ensuring you're not constantly preparing meals or bottles.

11. Give the Toddler a "Job" During Feeding
Involve the toddler in feeding the newborn by giving them a small task, like handing you a burp cloth or helping shake a bottle.
-Benefit: Keeps the toddler engaged and feeling helpful, reducing jealousy and distractions.

12. Use Distraction Tools for the Toddler
Set up a quiet activity (like coloring or puzzles) for the toddler to do while you feed the newborn.
-Benefit: Keeps the toddler occupied and calm while you focus on feeding the baby.

13. Prepare Easy-to-Eat Meals for the Toddler
Serve meals that don't require much help from you, like sandwiches, cut-up fruit, or scrambled eggs.
-Benefit: Allows the toddler to feed themselves with minimal assistance, giving you more time to focus on the newborn.

14. Set Up a Feeding Timer
Use a timer to set consistent intervals for toddler meals and newborn feedings to keep them on a regular schedule.
-Benefit: Creates a predictable routine for both, helping with meal planning and reducing chaos.

15. Have the Toddler Sit in a Child-Sized Chair
Use a child-sized table and chair for the toddler, so they can sit and eat independently while you feed the newborn.
-Benefit: Promotes self-sufficiency, making it easier to manage both feedings.

16. Encourage Independent Feeding for the Toddler
Teach your toddler to use a spoon, fork, or their hands to feed themselves while you attend to the newborn.
-Benefit: Builds confidence and independence in the toddler, making meal times smoother.

17. Give the Toddler a Drink During Newborn's Feeding Time
Offer the toddler milk, water, or a smoothie while you're feeding the newborn.
-Benefit: Keeps the toddler calm and content, reducing the need for your attention while the newborn is being fed.

18. Prepare Meals that Both Can Eat
As the newborn transitions to solids, prepare meals that both the toddler and baby can enjoy, like soft fruits, veggies, and purees.
-Benefit: Simplifies meal prep and reduces the need to make separate meals for each child.

19. Switch Between Breastfeeding and Bottle Feeding
Alternate between breastfeeding and bottle feeding the newborn, depending on what's easiest when managing the toddler's mealtime.
-Benefit: Allows for more flexibility and enables others to help with feeding while you attend to the toddler.

20. Stick to a Routine
Establish a consistent routine for feeding times for both the toddler and newborn, ensuring meals and feedings happen at the same time each day. -Benefit: Creates predictability and stability, making it easier to manage both children's needs at the same time.

Feeding toddlers and a newborn at the same time was a juggling act I had to master quickly. At first, the thought of it seemed overwhelming—how could I possibly meet everyone's needs at once without feeling like I was running in circles? But over time, I found a rhythm that worked for all of us.

My toddlers were used to their meal routine, so I made sure their plates were ready first. I would set them up with foods I knew they liked, like small portions of fruits, vegetables, and something filling, like whole grain toast or pasta. That way, they were happy and settled in their high chairs while I focused on the baby. For the newborn, I always made sure to plan feeding time when the toddlers were eating or occupied, so I could nurse or bottle-feed the baby without interruption.

One of the tricks that made things easier was having a high chair or bouncer close by so I could keep the baby nearby while I helped the toddlers eat. Some days were smoother than others—sometimes, the baby would fuss or one of the toddlers would spill something, but that's all part of the chaos of having little ones.

The benefit of feeding everyone at the same time was that we developed a routine where everyone ate together, which made mealtime more manageable. It also gave me a few moments of quiet once everyone was fed, and we could relax a bit before the next thing on the to-do list. Keeping snacks ready for the toddlers also helped—if the baby needed more attention, I knew my older ones could munch on something while I cared for the baby.

Eventually, I got into a groove where feeding all of them at once wasn't so stressful anymore. It became a part of our daily rhythm, and I felt accomplished knowing I could balance the needs of my growing family.

Handling Picky Eaters and Special Diets

1. Incorporate Variety Gradually
Introduce new foods slowly alongside familiar favorites.
-Benefit: Reduces resistance to trying new things and helps children become more comfortable with different textures and tastes.

2. Offer Choices
Let your child choose between two healthy options (e.g., carrots or cucumbers).
-Benefit: Empowers the child, making them more likely to eat without feeling forced.

3. Serve Small Portions
Start with small portions of new or disliked foods.
-Benefit: Reduces overwhelm and waste while encouraging them to try different foods.

4. Make Meals Fun
Use cookie cutters for sandwiches or arrange food into fun shapes.
-Benefit: Makes mealtime enjoyable and encourages even picky eaters to engage with their food.

5. Hide Veggies in Favorite Dishes
Puree vegetables into sauces, soups, or baked goods.
-Benefit: Ensures your child gets essential nutrients without realizing they're eating veggies.

6. Cook Together
Involve your child in meal prep by letting them wash vegetables or stir ingredients.
-Benefit: Increases curiosity and willingness to try foods they helped prepare.

7. Be a Role Model
Show enthusiasm for healthy foods by eating them yourself.
-Benefit: Encourages children to follow your lead, making them more likely
to try the same foods.

8. Create a Routine
Serve meals and snacks at consistent times each day.
-Benefit: Helps kids understand when to expect food, reducing random
snacking and picky behavior.

9. Respect Their Appetite
Avoid forcing your child to eat when they're not hungry.
-Benefit: Prevents negative associations with food and encourages children
to listen to their own hunger cues.

10. Incorporate "Safe" Foods
Always include one food you know your child likes at every meal.
-Benefit: Provides comfort and reassurance, increasing the likelihood they'll
try other items on the plate.

11. Introduce Foods Multiple Times
Offer new foods up to 10 times without pressure.
-Benefit: Studies show that repeated exposure increases acceptance of
new foods over time.

12. Avoid Becoming a Short-Order Cook
Stick to preparing one meal for the whole family instead of making separate
dishes for picky eaters.
-Benefit: Encourages children to eat what's served and reduces the stress
of managing different meals.

13. Pair New Foods with Familiar Ones
Serve new foods alongside something they already love.
-Benefit: Makes new foods seem less intimidating, increasing the chance
they'll take a bite.

14. Use Positive Reinforcement
Praise your child when they try new foods, even if they don't like them.
-Benefit: Reinforces positive eating behaviors without pressure, making
them more open to trying again.

15. Offer a Sensory Toy During Meals
Provide a small sensory toy (like a fidget or squishy) to keep their hands
busy while they eat.
-Benefit: Helps children who are easily distracted or need stimulation to
focus on their meal, making them more likely to sit through and eat.

16. Consult with a Pediatrician or Dietitian
If your child has special dietary needs, get expert advice on balanced meal
plans.
-Benefit: Ensures their nutritional requirements are met while
accommodating any restrictions.

17. Offer Dips or Sauces
Provide dips like hummus, yogurt, or nut butter to make foods more
appealing.
-Benefit: Adds flavor and excitement to vegetables or proteins, encouraging
children to eat more.

18. Incorporate Familiar Flavors into New Foods
Add familiar seasonings or flavors your child enjoys to new dishes.
-Benefit: Increases acceptance of new foods by making them taste similar
to something they already like.

19. Set Clear Meal Expectations
Establish rules like trying at least one bite or waiting until the meal is over
before leaving the table.
-Benefit: Creates structure without being overly restrictive, helping children
understand mealtime boundaries.

20. Use Food as Learning
Teach children about the benefits of different foods and how they help the body.
-Benefit: Encourages interest in healthy eating and empowers kids to make better food choices.

Handling picky eaters and special diets has always been a bit of a challenge in our household, but it's something I've learned to manage with patience and creativity. One of the first hurdles we faced was my daughter's lactose sensitivity. When we realized that dairy was causing her discomfort, we had to switch to lactose-free products and find alternatives that still provided the nutrients she needed. It was a bit of trial and error at first, but eventually, we found a balance that worked for her.

I've always been open with my kids about what's healthy and what's not. I believe that if they understand why we eat certain foods, they're more likely to embrace healthy eating. I'll never forget one day when we were in the grocery store, standing in a busy aisle, and my daughter loudly said, "We need to get vegetables because I like vegetables, and they are good for our bodies!" In that moment, I was beyond proud. All the talks we'd had about food and health were sinking in, and she was starting to make those choices on her own.

We've had a few funny moments along the way, too. Like the time when my kids told me they loved broccoli. I was so excited that I went to the store and bought a ton of frozen broccoli, thinking I was set for weeks. When I served it, though, they were less than thrilled, saying, "No, we like hard broccoli!" Turns out they meant fresh, uncooked broccoli, not the soft, steamed version I had made. Lesson learned!

One thing that helps make grocery shopping and mealtime special for them is letting them take turns grabbing items off the shelves. When they help choose the food, they feel more involved, and it becomes something they look forward to. When we sit down to eat, and they know they helped pick out the ingredients, they get excited about trying the food. It's such a simple way to make healthy eating fun for them and make them feel proud of their choices.

Through it all, I've found that handling picky eaters and special diets doesn't have to be a battle. It's about finding what works for each child, explaining the benefits of healthy foods, and making the process fun and engaging.

Chapter 11
Traveling with a Full House

Packing for All Ages

1. Make Detailed Packing Lists
Create a list for each child, categorizing by essentials (clothing, toiletries, comfort items).
-Benefit: Reduces the chance of forgetting anything and keeps you organized.

2. Pack as You Do Laundry
As clothes come out of the laundry, sort them directly into suitcases or bags.
-Benefit: Saves time by combining tasks and ensures you pack clean clothes.

3. Use Separate Bags for Different Items
Organize items like diapers, pump supplies, swimsuits, or toys into individual small bags.
-Benefit: Keeps things easily accessible and prevents clutter in the main bag.

4. Roll Clothes Instead of Folding
Roll clothes to save space and prevent wrinkles.
-Benefit: Maximizes suitcase space and keeps clothing neater.

5. Use Packing Cubes
Separate outfits and categories (socks, underwear, PJs) into packing cubes for each child.

-Benefit: Helps with quick unpacking and easy access to specific items.

6. Pack Each Child's Clothes in Ziploc Bags by Day
Label Ziploc bags with the day and pack an outfit for each child inside.
-Benefit: Saves time getting dressed and ensures all items are together.

7. Bring Extra Outfits
Pack one or two extra outfits per child, just in case of accidents or spills.
-Benefit: Prevents stress when things don't go as planned and you need a quick change.

8. Prepare a Separate Bag for Snacks
Designate a specific bag for snacks, drinks, and feeding supplies.
-Benefit: Keeps food organized and prevents spills on clothes or other items.

9. Pack a Portable Laundry Bag
Bring a small, collapsible bag for dirty clothes.
-Benefit: Keeps dirty laundry separate from clean clothes and ready for washing.

10. Include Comfort Items
Don't forget your kids' favorite blanket, stuffed toy, or pacifier.
-Benefit: Helps them feel secure and settle into new environments more easily.

11. Pre-Pack Toiletries in Travel-Sized Bottles
Use travel-sized containers for baby soap, lotion, and other toiletries.
-Benefit: Saves space and ensures you have just enough for the trip without overpacking.

12. Label Bags for Specific Purposes
Label small bags (diapers, pumping supplies, swimsuits) for easy identification.

-Benefit: Quick access to what you need without rummaging through everything.

13. Keep Essentials in a Carry-On
If flying, pack essentials like diapers, wipes, and a change of clothes in your carry-on.
-Benefit: Provides immediate access to necessary items in case of delays or lost luggage.

14. Pack for the Destination's Weather
Check the forecast and pack layers for variable weather.
-Benefit: Avoids over packing or being unprepared for changing temperatures.

15. Bring a First Aid Kit
Include band-aids, antiseptic wipes, medications, and any allergy supplies.
-Benefit: You'll be prepared for minor injuries or illnesses without hunting for supplies.

16. Use a Pumping Bag for Breastfeeding Supplies
Store your pump, bottles, and extra parts in a separate bag.
-Benefit: Keeps everything you need for feeding organized and sanitary.

17. Pack Swimwear in Waterproof Bags
Place swimsuits, goggles, and sunscreen in waterproof bags.
-Benefit: Keeps wet items from leaking onto other clothes.

18. Bring a Compact Stroller or Carrier
Pack a lightweight stroller or baby carrier for easy mobility.
-Benefit: Makes travel smoother and gives your arms a break.

19. Keep Important Documents Together
Gather travel documents, IDs, and tickets in a folder or zippered pouch.
-Benefit: Quick access when needed and reduces the risk of misplacing critical items.

20. Pack Entertainment for Different Ages
Include toys, books, or electronics suitable for each child's age.
-Benefit: Keeps kids entertained during travel, helping to avoid boredom and meltdowns.

When my kids were babies, it often felt like I was bringing the entire house with us every time we left. I'd pack everything I thought we might possibly need, from bouncers and swings to extra clothes, snacks, toys, and diapers—just in case. But as the trips went on, I started to notice something: a lot of the stuff I packed never even got touched. There would be outfits that stayed folded, toys that went ignored, and entire bags that I never even opened. That's when I realized I needed to figure out what we truly needed and what we could leave behind.

One of the biggest lifesavers for me was organizing everything into separate bags. I might not have remembered exactly where each item was, but I always knew which bag had what in it. I'd pack a diaper bag, a pumping bag, a snack bag, and so on, each one serving a specific purpose. It was such a relief because when I was juggling the kids, all I had to do was ask my husband to grab a specific bag—"Can you get the diaper bag, the blue one with the handles?"—and I knew we'd have what we needed without me scrambling around.

I also started making detailed lists before packing, which became another game-changer. The lists kept me organized and helped me focus on the essentials. It stopped me from over packing because I could check off items as I went and see if I was adding too much. It was comforting to have a clear plan and know exactly what I was bringing, rather than throwing things into the suitcase last minute and hoping for the best.

Looking back, learning what we really needed—versus what I thought we needed—made a world of difference. The bags became my system, and the lists helped me stay on track, making travel and outings with little ones much more manageable. And over time, I found our groove, packing only what was necessary, and I felt much more in control.

Making Travel Fun and Stress-Free

1. Pack a couple of interactive toys for each child
Choose toys like coloring books, or electronic games that engage them.
-Benefit: Keeps kids occupied and minimizes boredom.

2. Regulate water intake so they don't drink too much at once
Give children small sips of water at regular intervals rather than large
amounts at once.
-Benefit: Keeps them hydrated without causing frequent bathroom stops,
maintaining a balanced schedule.

3. Plan bathroom stops in advance and combine them with food breaks and
gas stops
Look up rest areas or restaurants along your route and stop for food and
bathroom breaks at the same time.
-Benefit: Saves time and reduces the number of stops.

4. Bring easy-to-eat snacks that are individually packaged or can be
portioned
Pre Pack snacks like crackers, fruits, and granola bars in small bags.
-Benefit: Reduces mess and makes snack time easier on the go.

5. Use containers to keep snacks organized
Pack snacks in reusable containers with lids or use snack boxes with
compartments.
-Benefit: Minimizes spills and keeps snacks fresh.

6. Arrange seating so children sit next to those they are least likely to fight
with
Seat siblings who get along better next to each other, or place a barrier like
a pillow between those who tend to argue.
-Benefit: Reduces arguments and creates a more peaceful environment.

7. Designate a toy bag for the car filled with engaging items
Fill a bag with toys specifically for the car, like small figurines, fidget toys, or books.
-Benefit: Keeps toys contained and easy to reach during the trip.

8. Have a separate snack bag specifically for car trips
Use a small cooler or bag to keep snacks accessible and organized.
-Benefit: Easy access to snacks without needing to unpack luggage.

9. Create a travel-friendly playlist with everyone's favorite music
Make a playlist ahead of time with songs each family member enjoys.
-Benefit: Boosts morale and makes the trip more enjoyable for everyone.

10. Pack extra clothes in case of spills or accidents
Keep a change of clothes in a separate, easy-to-reach bag for quick changes.
-Benefit: Reduces stress in case of accidents and avoids uncomfortable travel.

11. Use window shades to prevent sun glare and keep the car cool
Install stick-on window shades or bring blankets to cover the windows.
-Benefit: Keeps the car temperature comfortable and protects kids from harsh sunlight.

12. Bring blankets or travel pillows to make naps more comfortable
Pack small blankets and neck pillows for each child.
-Benefit: Promotes better naps and keeps children rested during the journey.

13. Schedule driving around nap times for quieter moments on the road
Plan to drive during times when your children typically nap.
-Benefit: Allows for quieter, uninterrupted driving while children rest.

14. Wear loose-fitting, easy clothes for both you and the kids
Choose comfortable, breathable clothing like leggings, soft shirts, or loose
pants for everyone.
-Benefit: Increases comfort during long periods of sitting and makes it
easier to handle quick stops for bathroom breaks or stretching.

15. Use a small trash bag or container for easy clean-up during the trip
Attach a small trash bag to the seat or use a container to collect garbage.
-Benefit: Keeps the car tidy and makes cleaning up easier at stops.

16. Pack an emergency kit with wipes, hand sanitizer, and bandages
Assemble a small kit with essential items for spills, cuts, or messes.
-Benefit: Prepares you for unexpected situations and helps maintain
hygiene.

17. Rotate toys during the trip to keep children's interest fresh
Swap out toys every hour or two to maintain engagement.
-Benefit: Prevents boredom and keeps children entertained longer.

18. Bring a tablet or device with educational apps for quiet entertainment
Download a few educational games or apps that children can enjoy quietly.
-Benefit: Provides a quiet, engaging activity that can also be educational.

19. Give older children responsibilities, like helping with snacks or music
selection
Assign small tasks like handing out snacks or choosing songs for older
kids.
-Benefit: Makes them feel involved and reduces boredom by giving them
purpose.

20. Bring a favorite stuffed animal or security object
Let each child bring a comforting item like a favorite toy or blanket.
-Benefit: Helps soothe anxiety and promotes relaxation during long trips.

Our road trips used to feel like a never-ending series of stops. In the beginning, we seemed to be pulling over every hour—whether for bathroom breaks, snacks, or just to let the kids stretch their legs. What should have been a six-hour drive easily turned into nine! It was exhausting for everyone, and I knew we had to do something differently.

Over time, I figured out a system that worked for us. Instead of stopping at random moments, I learned to combine our stops. When we pulled over for gas, I made sure everyone took a potty break, had a chance to move around, and grabbed a snack. It became our little routine, and we stuck to it. This way, we weren't constantly getting in and out of the car, and our trips became much smoother.

I also found a sweet spot for keeping the kids entertained. We packed interactive learning toys, and they took turns with them—switching every so often to keep things fresh. Whether it was a learning tablet that helped with letters or a book, it kept their minds engaged. But they each had their own special toy and blanket too. Lilly never goes anywhere without her boo boo bear, Hazen needs his favorite train, Lola loves her blanket, Skylar rotates between stuffies and Theo is cool with whatever his siblings don't take from him. Having their comfort items made them feel more settled, especially when the drive started to feel long.

As for screens, we reserve those for really long drives, and even then, only as a reward. "If you nap for a bit, you can watch something when you wake up," I would tell them. And sure enough, after a good rest, they earned their screen time. It worked like a charm—keeping the peace while still sticking to our no-screens-unless-necessary rule.

One of the biggest game changers, though, was rearranging the car seating. Lilly and Hazen, my two older ones, used to argue non stop when sitting next to each other. It was driving me crazy. Then, I had the idea to put the toddler between them. It was like magic! Now, not only do they argue less, but they actually help out with the toddler.

Road trips aren't perfect, but with a bit of planning and adjusting, they've become so much more manageable. And now, when we get to our destination, everyone's in a better mood, and I'm not completely wiped out!

Tips for Road Trips and Air Travel

1. Pack a collapsible stroller for airport or road rest stops
Use a lightweight, foldable stroller that's easy to transport and store.
-Benefit: Makes navigating airports or rest stops easier with young kids who tire quickly.

2. Bring a portable charger for devices
Ensure you have a fully charged power bank for phones, tablets, and other electronics.
-Benefit: Keeps devices powered during long trips, avoiding battery anxiety and ensuring entertainment is available.

3. Use packing cubes to organize luggage
Sort clothing and other essentials into separate packing cubes by category or person.
-Benefit: Saves space and makes it easier to find what you need without unpacking the entire suitcase.

4. Create a checklist of travel essentials
Write a list of must-have items and check them off as you pack.
-Benefit: Reduces the chance of forgetting important items, like passports, snacks, or chargers.

5. Download travel apps for navigation and updates
Use apps like Google Maps, Waze, or flight trackers to stay informed about routes or delays.
-Benefit: Keeps you updated on road conditions or flight changes, helping you adjust plans easily.

6. Pre-book transportation and accommodations
Reserve airport transfers, car rentals, or hotel stays ahead of time.
-Benefit: Saves time and ensures you have reliable transportation and
accommodations ready upon arrival.

7. Dress in layers
Wear easily removable layers like jackets or cardigans.
-Benefit: Allows you to adjust for temperature changes in airports,
airplanes, or during road trips.

8. Use noise-canceling headphones or earplugs
Bring noise-canceling headphones or earplugs for yourself and the kids.
-Benefit: Reduces background noise in cars or planes, helping with focus or
sleep.

9. Give each child their own backpack with essentials
Let each child carry a small backpack with their own toys, snacks, and a
water bottle.
-Benefit: Encourages independence and keeps their items organized and
easy to reach.

10. Have kids stretch and move at rest stops or layovers
Encourage kids to stretch, walk, or run around during breaks.
-Benefit: Helps them burn off energy and reduces restlessness during the
next leg of the journey.

11. Bring disposable or reusable bags for dirty clothes
Pack a few extra bags to separate dirty or wet clothes.
-Benefit: Keeps the rest of your luggage clean and organized.

12. Pack a first aid kit with motion sickness remedies
Include basic first aid items and motion sickness pills or bands.
-Benefit: Prepares you for minor illnesses or injuries during travel.

13. Check luggage policies for airlines or space in the car
Review your airline's baggage limits or car space before packing.
-Benefit: Avoids extra fees or frustration when trying to fit everything in.

14. Bring a refillable water bottle
Carry an empty water bottle through airport security and refill it once you
pass through.
-Benefit: Saves money and ensures everyone stays hydrated without
frequent purchases.

15. Pack non-liquid snacks for flights
Bring dry, non-liquid snacks that pass security, like nuts or granola bars.
-Benefit: Keeps hunger at bay without needing to rely on airplane food.

16. Use a baby carrier for air travel with infants
Bring a hands-free baby carrier to wear your baby through the airport or
during boarding.
-Benefit: Keeps your hands free for luggage or other tasks, and soothes the
baby during travel.

17. Keep all travel documents in a zippered pouch
Store passports, IDs, boarding passes, and other documents in one
easy-to-reach pouch.
-Benefit: Reduces stress by keeping all important items in one organized
place.

18. Bring small, new toys for surprise entertainment
Pack small toys or trinkets your child hasn't seen before and give them out
gradually.
-Benefit: Keeps children entertained with something new, minimizing
boredom.

19. Use a luggage tag with your contact info
Attach a luggage tag with your name, phone number, and email on all bags.
-Benefit: Increases the chances of recovering lost luggage quickly.

20. Bring a change of clothes in your carry-on
Always pack at least one full change of clothes for each person in the carry-on.
-Benefit: Prepares you in case of luggage delays, spills, or accidents during travel.

Our family trips were always full of little surprises, and not always the good kind—especially when it came to our devices dying at the worst possible moments. I remember one time, we were in the middle of nowhere, trying to find the next gas station, and of course, my phone died just when I needed to look up directions. It was the craziest timing! After that, I learned my lesson and never travel without a portable charger. It has saved us more times than I can count—whether it's for looking up something important or keeping the kids entertained on long car rides.

Another game changer was switching to a collapsible stroller. In the beginning, we started with a regular stroller, and let me tell you, it was a nightmare. It took up the entire trunk, and maneuvering it was like wrestling an alligator. That didn't last long. I finally upgraded to a collapsible one, it was a total lifesaver and cheaper. It fit everywhere, even in small spaces, and it made transporting the kids so much easier. If I had to focus on something else, I could just pop them in the stroller, and they'd stay in one spot. And if I was lucky, they might even take a nap, which gave me a much-needed break.

One of the best hacks I discovered for flying was bringing an empty water bottle for the kids. The first time I did it, my husband looked at me like I was crazy. "Why are you bringing trash onto the airport?" he asked, totally confused. But once we were past security and I filled it up, he was impressed. Not only did it save us from paying ridiculous prices for bottled water waiting for our flight, but it also meant the kids could drink from their own sippy cups without me having to share mine and deal with the inevitable backwash.

And the individual backpacks for the kids? Total genius. Each of them gets to pack their own bag with the toys they want, and for some reason, those same toys are way more exciting when they come out of their own backpacks rather than mine. It gives them a sense of responsibility and pride. Plus, having their own snacks in their bags somehow makes them taste better too! Traveling with kids is never easy, but with these little tricks, I've found a way to make it smoother. And every trip teaches me something new to add to my toolkit!

Chapter 12
Managing Screen Time for Different Ages

Setting Age-Appropriate Limits

1. Set daily screen time limits using timers
Use timers to mark the beginning and end of screen time.
-Benefit: Helps create structure, and children learn when it's time for other
activities.

2. Create screen-free zones in the home
Designate certain areas like bedrooms or the dining table as screen-free.
-Benefit: Encourages family bonding and supports healthy sleep habits.

3. Use parental controls on devices
Activate parental control settings on devices to filter content.
-Benefit: Protects young kids from inappropriate material while allowing
them to explore safely.

4. Encourage educational apps or shows
Provide access to apps or shows that promote learning and creativity.
-Benefit: Fosters curiosity and helps develop cognitive skills while keeping
screen time productive.

5. Establish a reward system for extra screen time
Create a system where children earn screen time by completing tasks like
chores or homework.
-Benefit: Motivates children to be responsible and teaches them to work for
rewards.

6. Model balanced screen habits
Show children how to balance screen time with other activities by doing the same yourself.
-Benefit: Kids learn healthy habits by observing and mimicking adult behavior.

7. Schedule daily physical play away from screens
Plan for outdoor or active playtime every day without screens.
-Benefit: Encourages physical development and reduces the risk of sedentary behavior.

8. Use only age-appropriate video games
Check game ratings and allow only those suitable for your child's age.
-Benefit: Ensures that kids engage with content that matches their developmental level.

9. Encourage both solo and shared screen activities
Provide time for independent play and also cooperative games with others.
-Benefit: Promotes social skills while offering time for self-entertainment.

10. Take frequent screen breaks
Incorporate regular breaks from screens to move around or play offline.
-Benefit: Prevents eye strain and promotes physical movement, supporting overall health.

11. Set an evening curfew for screen use
Establish a cutoff time for screens before bed.
-Benefit: Reduces exposure to blue light, leading to better sleep and relaxation before bedtime.

12. Co-watch or co-play games and shows
Participate in screen time with your child by watching or playing together.
-Benefit: Builds trust, offers bonding time, and allows for discussions about the content.

13. Rotate between screen time and non-screen activities
Alternate between using devices and doing things like reading, crafts, or playing outdoors.
-Benefit: Encourages balance and helps children appreciate a variety of activities.

14. Use screen time for family connection
Choose games or movies that everyone in the family can enjoy together.
-Benefit: Strengthens family bonds and creates positive memories involving screen use.

15. Offer creative offline alternatives
Provide toys, puzzles, or art supplies to engage kids in non-digital play.
Benefit: Encourages imagination, creativity, and critical thinking away from screens.

16. Introduce tech-free days or hours
Schedule entire days or blocks of time where no screens are allowed.
-Benefit: Encourages more active play, exploration, and family interaction without distractions.

17. Use screen time as a reward for physical activity
Allow extra screen time after kids engage in physical exercise or outdoor play.
-Benefit: Motivates children to stay active while still enjoying their favorite screen activities.

18. Encourage screen-free hobbies
Promote hobbies like drawing, building, or playing sports as alternatives to screen time.
-Benefit: Encourages the development of new skills and interests beyond digital entertainment.

19. Create a family tech schedule
Draft a schedule showing when screens can be used and when they should
be off.
-Benefit: Keeps the household on the same page and reduces conflicts
over screen use.

20. Set clear consequences for breaking screen time rules
Define consequences for when limits are ignored, such as reduced screen
time the next day.
-Benefit: Helps children respect boundaries and understand the importance
of following rules.

In our family, video games are something we all really enjoy, but we've worked hard to make sure they're more of a special treat than something we rely on. On the weekends, we love sitting down together to play, taking turns and cheering each other on. There's a lot of laughter and fun as we play our favorite games, whether it's racing, solving puzzles, or teaming up for an adventure. It's always a good time, and we've turned it into a great way to bond.

But as much as we love video games, the kids know that screen time isn't an everyday thing. It's not something they're entitled to, and it's definitely not something we do all day. There are no screens in the bedrooms at all—everything stays out in the living room, where we can enjoy it as a family. Even when we have screen time, it's balanced with other activities. We do so many things that don't involve screens, like building with blocks, crafting, reading books, or playing outside. The kids love exploring new activities, and it helps them realize there's more to do than just video games.

When it comes to movies, we usually have a family movie night while eating dinner, but even then, it's part of our routine and not something they expect all the time. They know when it's screen time and when it's not. In fact, they've gotten so used to our schedule that they don't even ask to earn screen time until it's the right time for it. They understand that screens are a privilege, and they've learned to enjoy them without feeling like they need to have them constantly.

This balance has really made a difference. Screen time is a fun part of our lives, but it's definitely not the only part, and I love that the kids have learned that too.

Earning Screen Time

1. Set Clear Rules
Establish simple, age-appropriate rules about when screen time is allowed and what needs to be done to earn it.
-Benefit: Helps children understand boundaries and expectations, making it easier to manage screen time.

2. Create a Routine
Set a daily routine where screen time is only available after chores or homework.
-Benefit: Encourages children to prioritize responsibilities before entertainment.

3. Use a Reward Chart
Make a chart where kids can earn screen time by completing tasks or good behavior.
-Benefit: Builds positive reinforcement and teaches the concept of earning rewards.

4. Teach Delayed Gratification
Let children wait until a specific time for screens, like after dinner or chores.
-Benefit: Instills patience and the value of working toward a reward.

5. Offer Non-Screen Rewards
Provide other rewards like stickers, small toys, or extra playtime alongside screen time.
-Benefit: Keeps the focus on a variety of incentives, not just screens.

6. Set Time Limits
Make sure children know exactly how long they can use screens once they earn it.
-Benefit: Helps them understand moderation and prevents excessive use.

7. Chore-Based Earning
Let children earn screen time by completing simple chores like picking up toys or setting the table.
-Benefit: Teaches responsibility and work ethic from a young age.

8. Encourage Outdoor Play First
Require some active playtime outside before screen time is allowed.
-Benefit: Promotes physical activity and helps balance screen time with outdoor play.

9. Educational Games as Bonus
Introduce educational apps or games that can be earned as a bonus after completing learning activities.
-Benefit: Combines learning with fun, showing children that screens can be educational.

10. Praise Effort, Not Just Results
Reward children for their effort in completing tasks or following rules, not just for the outcome.
-Benefit: Builds self-esteem and motivates children to keep trying.

11. Allow Kids to Choose Chores
Let them pick from a list of chores they can complete to earn screen time.
-Benefit: Increases their sense of control and responsibility.

12. Model Screen Time Balance
Show children that you also balance screen time with other activities like reading or exercising.
-Benefit: Kids learn by example, so they'll mimic healthy screen habits.

13. Use Screens as a Special Treat
Frame screen time as a special treat for weekends or after a big task is done.
-Benefit: Makes screens feel like a reward rather than an everyday right.

14. Combine Screen Time with Quiet Time
Reward screen time after quiet activities like reading or drawing.
-Benefit: Encourages creative play while still offering a screen-time reward.

15. Use Timers
Set a timer when screen time begins so they know exactly when it ends.
-Benefit: Provides structure and helps manage expectations.

16. Alternate Screen Time with Physical Activity
Create a system where they have to do a physical activity before earning
more screen time.
-Benefit: Balances physical activity with screen use, keeping them active.

17. Introduce a "No Screens Until" Rule
No screens until teeth are brushed, room is tidy, or toys are put away.
-Benefit: Teaches responsibility in maintaining their own space and habits.

18. Use Positive Reinforcement
Offer extra screen time for completing tasks without reminders or showing
great behavior.
-Benefit: Encourages self-discipline and motivates kids to do tasks
independently.

19. Involve Kids in the Process
Let them help set screen-time goals and limits, so they feel involved.
-Benefit: Encourages cooperation and gives them ownership over their
choices.

20. Stick to Consistency
Keep the rules and routine consistent, so kids know what to expect.
-Benefit: Establishes stability and makes it easier for children to follow the
rules.

In our household, video games are something the kids know they need to earn, but what surprised me most was when they stopped asking, "Can we play video games?" and started asking, "Can we earn video games?" It was such a shift in their mindset, and it made me proud to see that they understood the value of earning something, rather than expecting it to be given.

I like to keep things simple by offering only a few options for how they can earn their screen time. Each task is something they can work on and master, giving them a real sense of accomplishment when they finish. In the beginning, I helped guide them through these tasks, whether it was cleaning up their room, cleaning up the toys in the living room, or doing extra pages of homework. I showed them step by step how to do it, and at first, we did it together. But as time went on, I didn't have to show them anymore. They learned quickly, and as they grew older, the chores became a bit more challenging, matching their development and skill level.

The funny thing is, if they don't feel like playing video games on a particular day, they simply don't do the chore. There's no pressure—it's their choice. Sometimes they're totally okay with skipping a day, and I'm fine with that. But there are also moments when they don't want to do the task, and as much as it hurts my heart, I have to stick to my word. There are days when it's tough on me too. I want to give in when I see they're tired or frustrated, but I know consistency is important. I've learned that following through on what I say teaches them something far more valuable than just the chore itself.

They know the rules and know that I hold true to them. If they want to earn video game time, they've got to put in the effort. It's not about the games, really—it's about understanding responsibility and the satisfaction that comes from earning something. Even though it's tough sometimes, I've seen how much they've grown through this. And that's what makes it all worth it.

Finding Best Apps, Shows, and Games for Young Children

1. Age Appropriateness
Choose content designed specifically for your child's age range.
-Benefit: Ensures content is engaging without being too advanced or too simplistic, matching their cognitive and emotional development.

2. Educational Value
Look for media that incorporates learning into fun activities or stories.
-Benefit: Encourages development in areas like literacy, math, problem-solving, and social skills while keeping kids entertained.

3. Positive Role Models
Pick shows or games that feature characters who exhibit good behavior and positive traits like kindness, teamwork, and empathy.
-Benefit: Reinforces values like cooperation, compassion, and respect.

4. Interactive Elements
Seek apps or games that require active participation, like solving puzzles or making choices.
-Benefit: Stimulates critical thinking and creativity, engaging children in active learning instead of passive consumption.

5. Parental Controls
Find apps or streaming services with robust parental controls to manage content and screen time.
-Benefit: Helps create a safe and manageable environment for children to explore media.

6. Diverse Representation
Look for content that showcases a variety of cultures, backgrounds, and experiences.
-Benefit: Fosters inclusivity, broadens understanding, and promotes empathy for people different from themselves.

7. No In-App Purchases
Choose apps that don't encourage in-app purchases or extra fees.
-Benefit: Prevents accidental purchases and keeps the experience stress-free for parents.

8. Minimal Ads
Select content with little to no advertising.
-Benefit: Reduces distractions and ensures a more focused and safer experience for young children.

9. Engaging Music and Sounds
Opt for media with pleasant music and sound effects that enhance the learning experience.
-Benefit: Stimulates auditory learning and makes the experience more immersive and enjoyable.

10. Offline Play Options
Look for apps and games that can be used offline for trips or areas without Wi-Fi.
-Benefit: Keeps children engaged during travel or in locations with poor internet connectivity.

11. Short, Digestible Episodes or Activities
Choose media with brief episodes or short, easy-to-complete activities.
-Benefit: Maintains attention span and makes it easier for young children to stay focused.

12. Parent Reviews
Research apps, shows, and games by reading reviews from other parents.
-Benefit: Provides insights into real-world usability, potential issues, and overall satisfaction from a trusted source.

13. Customization and Adaptability
Find apps or games that allow personalization, such as adapting difficulty levels or setting preferences.
-Benefit: Enables content to grow with the child's development, keeping them challenged but not overwhelmed.

14. Learning Progress Tracking
Look for apps that track your child's progress or provide feedback on their learning.
-Benefit: Allows parents to monitor development and understand what skills their child is mastering.

15. Hands-On Learning
Choose media that encourages hands-on interaction or physical play, such as games with puzzles or building elements.
-Benefit: Helps develop fine motor skills and cognitive abilities through active, tactile engagement.

16. Offline Play Recommendations
Opt for media that promotes offline activities, such as crafts or outdoor play inspired by the content.
-Benefit: Encourages balance between screen time and physical activities, promoting overall well-being.

17. Storytelling and Imagination
Look for apps and shows that inspire creativity through storytelling and imaginative play.
-Benefit: Helps children develop language, emotional understanding, and the ability to think creatively.

18. Progressive Difficulty
Select games or apps that gradually increase in difficulty.
-Benefit: Keeps children engaged by challenging them at the right level, fostering a sense of accomplishment.

19. Family Involvement
Choose media that encourages family interaction, like multiplayer games or
co-viewing.
-Benefit: Strengthens family bonds and allows for shared learning
experiences.

20. Certification and Awards
Look for apps or media with endorsements from educational organizations
or industry awards.
-Benefit: Provides assurance of high-quality, developmentally appropriate
content.

I've always been pretty picky about what my kids watch, and I'm okay with others having cable, but for us, not having it makes it much easier to control what they see. I realized how important this was when my first daughter was still young. One day, she screamed at me and stomped her feet in frustration—behavior that was completely out of character for her. It caught me off guard because she had never done anything like that before. A few days later, I was watching one of my favorite childhood movies with her, and it hit me—there was literally a whole scene, even a song, about how to throw a fit! I realized that she had been mimicking what she saw in the movie.

From that point on, I made a rule: I always watch anything new first to make sure it's up to my standards. It's not just about whether the content is "good," but about the kind of behavior it models. I want to be sure they're absorbing positive messages instead of learning how to throw tantrums or disrespect people.

When it comes to apps, I take the same approach. I like to download an app and test it out myself before letting the kids use it. There are so many good educational apps out there, but some have way too many ads or hidden charges. I'm not a fan of that. I prefer apps that can be played offline and don't have pop-up ads. If there are any ads, I'd rather they be sent to my email than risk my kids accidentally clicking on something.

One of the activities my kids really enjoy is following along with art tutorials. We do it together, and they think it's so cool that I join in with them. I also use some apps and videos for homeschooling, and they love it because it makes learning feel fun and interactive. As they get better at things, I either adjust the settings to make it more challenging or delete the app altogether and find something new.

We also use meditation apps, especially for sensory time, bedtime, and even timeouts. I like to record the meditations on a simple device so they don't get distracted by using their tablets or phones. It helps them calm down without the temptation of playing games or watching videos instead. It's all about finding that balance between what's fun, educational, and appropriate for them, and I'm glad we've found a system that works for us.

Finding Moments for Yourself

1. Set a Daily Quiet Time
Establish a quiet time for everyone, even if it's just 15 minutes. Use this time to read, meditate, or just breathe.
-Benefits: Helps reset your mind and reduces stress.

2. Wake Up Earlier
Get up slightly earlier to enjoy a quiet cup of coffee or stretch before the day starts.
-Benefits: Gives you a peaceful start, making the day feel less rushed.

3. Delegate Tasks to Family Members
Assign small tasks to your partner or older kids. Letting go of some responsibilities frees up time.
-Benefits: Lightens your load and teaches children responsibility.

4. Use Nap Time for Yourself
Instead of doing chores, take a nap or do something relaxing while the kids sleep.
-Benefits: Recharges your energy and reduces burnout.

5. Incorporate Short Exercises
Do 5-10 minutes of stretching, yoga, or walking during the day, even while kids play.
-Benefits: Increases energy and improves mental clarity.

6. Practice Mindful Breathing
Take a few moments throughout the day to practice deep breathing, especially during stressful times.
-Benefits: Lowers anxiety and helps calm your mind.

7. Create a Simple Skincare Routine
Take 5 minutes in the morning or evening for skincare. It's a small act that can feel refreshing.
-Benefits: Promotes self-care and boosts self-confidence.

8. Listen to Music or a Podcast
Put on your favorite playlist or listen to a short podcast while cooking or cleaning.
-Benefits: Adds joy to routine tasks and engages your mind.

9. Set Boundaries with Screen Time
Limit screen time for your kids so you can use that time to enjoy a book or focus on your hobbies.
-Benefits: Gives you uninterrupted moments and encourages family balance.

10. Schedule a Regular Break
Arrange for a family member or babysitter to give you a short break once a week.
-Benefits: Provides time to rest or pursue hobbies, renewing your energy.

11. Join a Parenting Group
Engage in a supportive community where you can share experiences and seek advice.
-Benefits: Reduces feelings of isolation and offers a support network.

12. Treat Yourself to Something Small
Every now and then, buy yourself something small—a favorite snack, coffee, or book.
-Benefits: Provides little moments of joy that lift your mood.

13. Use a Planner or Journal
Write down your thoughts, schedule, or goals. Organizing your day helps clear mental clutter.
-Benefits: Boosts productivity and reduces overwhelm.

14. Take a Walk Alone
If possible, go for a short walk by yourself to enjoy fresh air and quiet time.
-Benefits: Improves mental clarity and gives you a sense of peace.

15. Do a Quick Declutter
Spend 10 minutes decluttering a space. A clean area can make you feel more organized and calm.
-Benefits: Creates a more peaceful environment and reduces stress.

16. Have a Weekly Self-Care Ritual
Schedule a dedicated time for self-care, such as a bath, face mask, or reading time.
-Benefits: Prioritizes your well-being and serves as a relaxing break.

17. Ask for Help
Reach out to family or friends when you're feeling overwhelmed. Sometimes just talking helps.
-Benefits: Relieves stress and gives you emotional support.

18. Limit Multitasking
Focus on one task at a time, even if it's small. Juggling too much can increase stress.
-Benefits: Improves focus and reduces feeling overwhelmed.

19. Find Time for a Hobby
Spend 10-15 minutes doing something you love—painting, knitting, gardening—whatever brings you joy.
-Benefits: Nurtures your passions and offers a creative outlet.

20. Unplug for an Hour
Disconnect from your phone or screens for an hour. Use that time to be fully present or relax.
-Benefits: Reduces digital stress and encourages mindfulness.

When I first started waking up before my kids, it wasn't a grand plan. It began with just five minutes of quiet time to myself—nothing extravagant. But over time, I began to wake up earlier, gradually building it up to a couple of hours. There's something almost magical about those early hours, the peace that comes when the house is still and my brain isn't preoccupied with the endless to-do lists or worries of the day. During that time, I can think more clearly, focus, and actually get things done.

When I have those moments of downtime—like waiting for my toddler to finish up on the potty or keeping an eye on the kids in the bath—I sneak in a quick workout. They think I'm being silly but I know setting a healthy example is important. Every little bit helps, whether it's a set of squats or stretching while I'm waiting. I even make mindful decisions in how I move throughout the day, like picking up toys with a proper squat or switching sides when holding one of my little ones to keep my body balanced. Even small habits, like not finishing off their plates and being mindful of my own portions, make a big difference over time.

I always keep a running list of the things I want to accomplish. I don't set out to finish it all in one day—it's more about making progress, even if it's just 1%. That little bit adds up, and eventually, everything gets done without feeling overwhelmed. It's all about building habits, taking small steps, and trusting the process.

Each day, I make sure to listen to at least one self-help video and focus on books that offer solutions to what I might be struggling with. There's always an answer out there, and I try to find it. Before holidays, or if life feels too chaotic, I'll do a declutter and give things away to those who need them. It's amazing how clearing out physical space helps with mental clarity too.

Breathing exercises have become a part of my routine, but it wasn't always that way. Before kids, those breaths might have been replaced by muttered bad words when things got frustrating. Now, I make a conscious choice to breathe deeply instead. I even teach my kids how to use breathing techniques, and it's the sweetest thing when I see them take a deep breath on their own to calm down.

It's a mix of mindfulness, small daily habits, and giving myself grace that keeps me grounded. And somehow, through it all, things get done without me feeling like I'm drowning in the chaos.

Mental Health Tips for Handling Stress

1. Set Realistic Expectations
Accept that you can't do everything perfectly.
-Benefit: Reduces feelings of failure and frustration, helps manage stress
levels.

2. Take Breaks, Even Short Ones
Step away for a few minutes during overwhelming moments.
-Benefit: Refreshes your mind, giving you patience and perspective.

3. Develop a Simple Daily Routine
Create a routine for yourself and your kids that includes downtime.
-Benefit: Brings structure, making the day feel more manageable and less
chaotic.

4. Practice Gratitude
Reflect on small moments of joy each day.
-Benefit: Shifts focus from stress to positive experiences, improving mood.

5. Prioritize Self-Care
Schedule time for activities you enjoy, even if it's just 10 minutes.
-Benefit: Helps you feel more balanced and less overwhelmed.

6. Use Positive Affirmations
Repeat affirmations like "I am doing my best" when stressed.
-Benefit: Boosts confidence and reduces negative self-talk.

7. Limit Social Media
Set boundaries for how much time you spend online.
-Benefit: Reduces comparison, which can contribute to stress and
self-doubt.

8. Find Time for Physical Activity
Incorporate quick exercises or stretches throughout the day.
-Benefit: Boosts endorphins, reducing stress and improving mood.

9. Stay Hydrated and Eat Well
Make sure to drink water and eat regular, nutritious meals.
-Benefit: Physical well-being directly impacts mental health, keeping you energized.

10. Get Enough Sleep
Create a consistent sleep routine and rest when you can.
-Benefit: Sleep restores your energy and improves your ability to handle stress.

11. Laugh Often
Watch something funny, or find humor in everyday parenting moments.
-Benefit: Laughter is a natural stress reliever, boosting mood instantly.

12. Create Personal Boundaries
Establish times when you can focus on yourself, even if it's brief.
-Benefit: Protects your mental space and helps you recharge.

13. Practice Mindfulness
Stay present during everyday tasks, focusing on what's in front of you.
-Benefit: Reduces anxiety by focusing on the here and now, not future worries.

14. Use "Quiet Time" for Relaxation
Set up quiet activities for your children while you relax.
-Benefit: Gives you a moment to rest, even with kids nearby.

15. Celebrate Small Wins
Acknowledge small achievements, whether it's finishing laundry or calming a tantrum.
-Benefit: Builds a sense of accomplishment, boosting mental resilience.

16. Let Go of Guilt
Forgive yourself for not being perfect.
-Benefit: Frees you from unnecessary stress and promotes a kinder
self-image.

17. Simplify Your To-Do List
Focus on the most important tasks and let go of perfectionism.
-Benefit: Reduces overwhelm and helps you focus on what truly matters.

18. Create a Calm Space
Set aside a space in your home where you can relax, even if it's just a
corner.
-Benefit: Provides a retreat for when you need a mental break.

19. Limit Overcommitment
Be selective about activities and commitments outside of home life.
-Benefit: Avoids burnout by ensuring you're not taking on too much.

20. Celebrate "Me Time" Without Guilt
Take time for yourself without feeling guilty—whether it's a bath, a walk, or
quiet reading time.
-Benefit: Reinforces self-care as a necessary part of being a healthy and
balanced parent.

I used to feel incredibly guilty about doing things for myself, and to be honest, I still feel that way sometimes, just not as much. It's like that classic example: if your child falls into a pool and you don't know how to swim, you'll only make things worse by jumping in. You have to learn how to swim first, so you can be there to help them. That might sound extreme, but the same applies to taking care of yourself. If you're feeling sad, run-down, or overwhelmed, how are you going to show your kids the good in the world? Eventually, they'll absorb what you're putting out. They grow up watching, and you have to model the behavior you want them to see.

One of the ways I started doing things for myself was to combine self-care with time spent with my kids. My daughter and I get our nails done together now. It's a little treat for both of us. In the past, I would go to the store and only shop for them—everything for the kids, never for me. Now, I make sure to get at least one small thing that brings me joy, even if it's something simple like chocolate. And yes, I've taken to hiding little bits of chocolate around the house for those stressful moments when I need a quick pick-me-up.

Something that helped me snap out of tough times, especially when I had postpartum depression, was practicing gratitude. I learned this trick during that difficult period. Whenever I felt overwhelmed or sad, I forced myself to say five things out loud that I was grateful for. If that didn't lift my spirits, I'd keep saying more until I felt just a little better. Over time, it got easier. I didn't need to say as many things to find that spark of joy, and eventually, I could just say them in my head. But during those dark moments, I had to push myself to focus on gratitude. It was my way of rewiring my brain to see the positives.

Science backs up this practice too. When you focus on gratitude, it releases dopamine and serotonin—two neurotransmitters that improve mood and make you feel happier. Gratitude actually changes the brain by encouraging the production of these "feel-good" chemicals, helping to reduce stress and anxiety. It's not just a mindset trick; it's a brain-altering practice that makes a real difference in how you feel over time.

During their quiet time, I used to rush around trying to get everything done. I'd overwork myself to the point where I'd be completely drained by the time they woke up, and that would leave me feeling even more stressed. But now, I make sure to plan those moments better. I set aside a little down time for myself in between the to-dos, and it has made a world of difference.

Lowering my expectations has also been key. I had to remind myself that kids are just that—kids. My children are generally well-behaved, so when they do act out, it can catch me off guard. But instead of getting upset, I take a step back and remember that they're still learning. I'd much rather them jump on the couch playing "hot lava" than sit perfectly still all the time. The couch will survive, or eventually, we'll get a new one. Yes, the carpet gets messy, and things sometimes break, but I try to focus on what matters.

I don't want my kids to be scared of getting in trouble; I want them to learn how to solve problems. Sometimes that means they try to fix something on their own and come to me for help when it's too late. It can be heartbreaking, like when my son was four and accidentally broke his fishing pole. Instead of freaking out, he asked me for glue to fix it. I was so proud that he took responsibility and stayed calm, even if I couldn't actually fix it in the end.

Creating a calm space is something I've had to work on too. I remember being in the thick of things when my husband and I would sit on the kitchen floor to eat dinner while the kids were in the living room. If we went into the living room with them, they'd whine and ask for our food, even though it was the same as theirs. But if they couldn't see us, just a few feet away behind the counter, they were perfectly content. That spot behind the counter became my little hideout. Even today, when I need a moment, I sit there where I can see them, but they can't see me. It's a tiny retreat, but it makes a difference.

Balancing Your Needs with Your Family's

1. Set Boundaries with Family Time
Establish clear times when you focus solely on family and times when you focus on yourself. Communicate this with your family so everyone understands.
-Benefits: Allows for uninterrupted personal time while also giving your family undivided attention, reducing stress and fostering better relationships.

2. Delegate Household Tasks
Share responsibilities with your spouse and children. Assign age-appropriate chores to kids and make it a collaborative effort.
-Benefits: Lessens your burden and teaches your kids responsibility and teamwork.

3. Use Time Blocks for Personal & Family Time
Plan specific times of day for family activities and separate times for personal activities (e.g., reading, hobbies). Use a calendar to block off these times.
-Benefits: Ensures a structured day, helping you fit in personal time without guilt or disruption to family needs.

4. Practice "No Guilt" Self-Care
Remind yourself that taking care of your needs is essential for your well-being and your ability to care for your family. Reframe self-care as necessary, not selfish.
-Benefits: Reduces burnout and makes you more emotionally and mentally available for your family.

5. Create a Morning Routine That Benefits Everyone
Wake up early, do something for yourself (meditation, exercise), and then
shift into preparing for the family's day. This helps you feel accomplished
before family demands kick in.
-Benefits: Starting the day on your terms reduces stress and makes it
easier to transition into family-focused activities.

6. Simplify Your Schedule
Cut out unnecessary activities or commitments that are adding stress and
not serving your family or personal needs. Focus on what matters most.
-Benefits: A simpler schedule allows for more quality time with your family
and gives you breathing room for personal moments.

7. Embrace "Good Enough" Parenting
Accept that you can't do everything perfectly. Focus on being present and
doing your best rather than striving for perfection.
-Benefits: Reduces anxiety and lets you enjoy your time with your family
more, without the pressure of perfection.

8. Prioritize One-on-One Time with Each Child
Schedule short, focused time with each child during the week, even if it's
just 10-15 minutes of undivided attention.
-Benefits: Strengthens your bond with each child, ensures they feel special,
and gives you a clear sense of accomplishment as a parent.

9. Create a "You-Only" Space
Designate a space in your home where you can retreat for a few moments
of peace when needed—this could be a corner of a room, a nook, or even
a closet.
-Benefits: Having a physical space that's just for you helps clear your mind
and recharge, so you can return to your family with more energy and
patience.

10. Set Weekly Family Goals Together
Sit down with your family and decide on weekly goals (e.g., going to the park, eating dinner together). Make it a family project.
-Benefits: Involving everyone in planning balances family needs while allowing you to stay on track with your personal goals.

11. Limit Social Media & Screen Time
Set boundaries on your use of social media and electronics. Dedicate certain hours of the day or specific times to be completely offline.
-Benefits: Less distraction means more time for personal growth and meaningful family interaction.

12. Set Up Family Traditions
Create simple family traditions (Sunday movie night, weekend nature walks) that help you all bond without feeling like you need to fill every free moment with productivity.
-Benefits: Strengthens family relationships, creates lasting memories, and gives you set times to relax with your family.

13. Have a "Reset Day" for You and Your Family
Designate one day (or a few hours) each week where you and your family just relax—no chores, no running errands, just being together or alone as needed.
-Benefits: Gives everyone a mental break, allowing you to recharge and be more present in your roles afterward.

14. Create a Family Meal Prep Routine
Involve your family in meal prepping for the week. Assign tasks based on skill level and do it together, so you can save time during busy weeknights.
-Benefits: Saves you time and energy while also teaching your kids life skills and making family time more productive.

15. Use Waiting Times for Personal Time
During those pockets of waiting (like school pick-up or kids' extracurricular activities), take a moment to do something you enjoy, like reading or listening to an audiobook.
-Benefits: Turns downtime into valuable "me time," which can be hard to come by with young kids.

16. Combine Your Interests with Family Time
Find activities that overlap with both your interests and your family's, like outdoor walks, art projects, or gardening.
-Benefits: Strengthens family bonds while allowing you to engage in activities that also bring you joy.

17. Practice Saying "No" to Unnecessary Requests
Learn to say no to obligations or social engagements that don't benefit your family or personal life.
-Benefits: Protects your time and energy, leaving you with more space to focus on what truly matters.

18. Implement a Family Quiet Hour
Set aside one hour a day where everyone in the household engages in quiet activities (reading, drawing, etc.). Use this time for yourself as well.
-Benefits: Provides a regular break from the chaos, giving you a chance to recharge while fostering creativity and calm for your kids.

19. Plan a Personal or Family Staycation
Every few months, plan a mini-break for yourself or the family. Even if it's just a weekend at home with no plans, treat it like a vacation—disconnect from your regular routine.
-Benefits: Helps reset your energy and mental state, making you better able to handle both personal and family needs afterward.

20. Keep a Journal for Both Family and Self
Keep a journal where you can track family milestones and accomplishments as well as personal goals and reflections.
-Benefits: This practice gives you a sense of achievement, helping you balance what's important for both your family and yourself while offering perspective on your progress.

It used to feel like the kids were taking over the whole house, every room filled with toys, noise, and chaos. While we loved our children's energy and seeing them explore, there came a point where we needed to reclaim some space for ourselves. So, we made a decision—our room and the kitchen would become adults-only zones. The rest of the house could be for the kids to enjoy, but those two rooms would give us the peace and personal space we needed.

Having these boundaries has been a game-changer. Our bedroom became a sanctuary, a place where we could retreat and unwind without stepping on Legos or having to negotiate snack-time requests. The kitchen, too, became a calm, organized space where we could prepare meals and connect as a couple without little hands grabbing at every plate. This arrangement made the rest of the house feel like a safe, kid-friendly zone where they could roam and play freely. With our personal space carved out, I became more comfortable with the kids owning the rest of the house. They had their freedom, and we had our peace.

We're also big into family traditions, which play a huge role in maintaining balance and connection. These little rituals and routines—whether it's Friday movie night, weekend pancake breakfasts, or holiday traditions—give our family something to look forward to. They provide structure and routine, but also a sense of security and excitement. The kids know what's coming, and that makes everything feel more grounded. Plus, these traditions deepen our family bond. There's something magical about seeing your kids' eyes light up, knowing that they treasure these moments just as much as we do.

Speaking of weekends, I've learned to reserve them mostly for relaxation. It's time for the whole family to unwind, especially when Dad's home. We use that time to connect, whether it's lounging around in our PJs, taking walks together, or just playing. Of course, sometimes we do need to get things done depending on how the week went, but we make sure to keep the balance between productivity and quality family time. This keeps the weekends from feeling like a marathon and lets us focus on the moments that matter.

It was hard, but I also made a conscious effort to step back from social media. I realized I was constantly comparing myself to other moms, seeing these perfectly staged photos, and feeling like I wasn't measuring up. But once I stepped back, I reminded myself that I shouldn't be comparing my life to anyone else's—especially not to curated images. The only person I need to compare myself to is who I was yesterday. That shift in mindset has been incredibly freeing.

Setting game plans to achieve my goals has become a huge part of my life. I've always been one to set goals for myself, but I realized that I was overlooking the importance of doing the same for my kids. Sure, we focus on the usual milestones—walking, talking, potty training—but setting smaller, more intentional goals with them has been life-changing. I sit down with them and we make achievable goals together. The way their eyes light up when we talk about these goals is incredible. It gives them something to work toward, but also teaches them the value of good habits and working to achieve something. It's up to me to help guide them through the process, because they're still kids and learning. But I know these lessons will serve them well for years to come.

Creating this balance between personal space, family traditions, and teaching my kids about good habits and life lessons has brought so much harmony to our home. It's about finding that sweet spot where everyone's needs are met—mine, my husband's, and the kids'. By making space for ourselves, we've created more room for joy, growth, and connection as a family.

Chapter 14
Keeping Your Relationship Strong

Maintaining Connection Amid Parenthood

1. Treat Each Other with Kindness, No Matter What
Even when you're both in the thick of parenting or disagreements, commit
to treating each other kindly, focusing on words of encouragement.
-Benefit: Creates a foundation of respect and affection, even during tough
times, which strengthens your bond.

2. Call or Text Just to Say 'I Love You'
Send a simple message or call in the middle of the day to remind your
partner you're thinking of them.
-Benefit: Reinforces emotional intimacy and keeps the connection alive
throughout the day.

3. Hold a Hug for Longer Than 10 Seconds
When you hug, hold each other for at least 10 seconds. This duration
boosts the release of oxytocin, the bonding hormone.
-Benefit: Deepens physical and emotional connection, helping both
partners feel more grounded and loved.

4. Hold a Kiss for Longer Than 5 Seconds
Instead of a quick peck, kiss your partner for at least 5 seconds to show
intentional affection.
-Benefit: Increases emotional intimacy and strengthens the romantic aspect
of the relationship.

5. Know the Signs of Your Partner's Stress
Pay attention to when your partner seems overwhelmed, whether it's
through their body language or tone.
-Benefit: Recognizing stress early allows you to offer support before things
escalate, showing that you're attuned to their needs.

6. Know What Brings Your Partner Joy
Be mindful of their favorite hobbies, foods, or activities, and encourage them to indulge in those things regularly.
-Benefit: Supporting your partner's happiness helps them feel valued and appreciated, deepening your connection.

7. Do Small Acts of Kindness 'Just Because'
Leave a sweet note, make their favorite snack, or take over a chore without being asked.
-Benefit: These small gestures show thoughtfulness and remind your partner that you're thinking of them even amidst busy days.

8. Set Aside Time for Just the Two of You
Schedule a regular date night, even if it's a simple meal after the kids go to bed.
-Benefit: Prioritizing time alone helps keep the romantic and personal connection alive, beyond just parenting together.

9. Express Gratitude Daily
Take time each day to thank your partner for something specific they've done.
-Benefit: Feeling appreciated boosts both partners' well-being and reinforces positive behavior.

10. Compliment Each Other Often
Offer sincere compliments, whether about their appearance, parenting skills, or something they did that day.
-Benefit: Builds confidence and strengthens emotional intimacy, reminding your partner they are seen and valued.

11. Be Physically Affectionate Throughout the Day
Simple touches like holding hands, back rubs, or quick kisses throughout
the day show ongoing affection.
-Benefit: Keeps the connection strong, reminding you both of your bond
even during busy days.

12. Talk About Your Day, Even If It's Brief
Take a few minutes at the end of the day to check in and share highlights or
struggles from your day.
-Benefit: Keeps open communication flowing and helps you stay in tune
with each other's lives outside of parenting.

13. Share Your Goals and Dreams
Regularly talk about long-term goals and aspirations, both individually and
as a couple.
-Benefit: Helps align your vision for the future and reinforces the sense of
being on the same team.

14. Laugh Together
Find moments to share a joke, watch a funny show, or reflect on something
humorous that happened.
-Benefit: Laughter is a powerful way to relieve stress and strengthen the
bond between partners.

15. Celebrate Small Wins
Acknowledge and celebrate achievements, even small ones, like getting
through a tough week with the kids.
-Benefit: Celebrating together builds positivity and reinforces a supportive
partnership.

16. Check In About Feelings Regularly
Ask your partner how they're really feeling, beyond the surface-level daily
check-ins.
-Benefit: Creates a deeper emotional connection by encouraging
vulnerability and open communication.

17. Plan and Dream for Future Adventures
Talk about trips you'd like to take, projects you'd like to start, or anything exciting on the horizon.
-Benefit: Keeps the excitement alive in the relationship and gives you both something to look forward to.

18. Make Time for Intimacy
Prioritize physical intimacy, even if it requires scheduling it amid your busy lives.
-Benefit: Helps maintain a deep physical and emotional bond, preventing feelings of disconnect.

19. Share Responsibilities
Divide household and parenting duties fairly, and occasionally take on your partner's tasks to give them a break.
-Benefit: Promotes teamwork and reduces feelings of resentment that can build when one partner feels overwhelmed.

20. Support Each Other's Personal Growth
Encourage your partner's hobbies, interests, or career goals, offering to help make time for them.
-Benefit: Allows both partners to grow as individuals, which in turn strengthens the relationship as each person feels fulfilled.

My husband and I have been madly in love for over ten years, and despite all that we've been through, our relationship has only grown stronger. He's the one person I can be around constantly without ever getting tired of him. We have a connection that doesn't need words—just being near each other is enough to feel at peace. Even when we have downtime apart, we call each other. Sometimes we don't even talk much; just having him on the other end of the line brings me comfort. There have been countless times when I've called him, venting about a hard day, and he shows up with kettle corn and hot chocolate, as if he knows exactly what I need.

Whenever I'm out shopping, I always pick up a Reese's for him. He isn't big into gifts, his love language is touch. So, I make sure to hold his hand, scratch his back, or give him little touches throughout the day, just to let him know he's loved. It's not hard for me to do because making him happy brings me so much joy. My love language, on the other hand, is time, and he makes sure to spend as much time with us as possible. Honestly, I'd rather be with him in a cardboard box than live in an empty mansion without him.

One of the best parts of our relationship is how much we laugh together. We have the same sense of humor, and some of the jokes we share would probably make other people think we're weird, but to us, they're hilarious. I think that's what keeps us sane, especially when we're in the thick of the craziness that life throws at us.

No matter what, we always greet each other warmly and say goodbye, even if we're upset. It's important because even when we're angry or frustrated, we still love each other deeply. I know I can be guilty of getting short-tempered when the house is messy, and he always notices. Without saying a word, he starts cleaning, and suddenly, it feels like a weight has been lifted off of me. He knows me so well that sometimes he can sense what I need before I even realize it.

Both of us have struggled with poor self-image at different times, but we do a great job of boosting each other up and holding each other accountable.

Before we met, I used to spend hours on my hair and makeup, but over the years, he's helped me feel comfortable in my own skin. He makes me feel beautiful just as I am, and I try to do the same for him.

Through all the ups and downs, we've learned how to be each other's biggest support. Our love has grown stronger with every challenge, and there's no one else I'd rather go through life with.

Date Nights at Home

1. Wake Up Before the Kids
Set your alarm for 30 minutes to an hour before the kids wake up. Spend
this time connecting over coffee or talking quietly.
-Benefit: Starting the day together helps build connection and sets a
positive tone for the rest of the day.

2. Establish a Regular Bedtime for the Kids
Set a consistent bedtime routine for the kids so they are asleep early
enough for you to have time with your partner.
-Benefit: Having quiet time at the end of the day allows you to reconnect
without distractions, strengthening your relationship.

3. Cuddle During Family Time
Sit together on the couch during family movie night or playtime, and take
moments to hug or cuddle in front of the kids.
-Benefit: Being affectionate shows the kids a positive example of love and
connection, while also building closeness between you and your partner.

4. Cook Dinner Together After the Kids Are Asleep
Wait until the kids are in bed and then cook a simple or special dinner
together, making it a fun, interactive activity.
-Benefit: Cooking together can be a shared experience that fosters
teamwork and adds an element of fun to your evening.

5. Have a Themed Movie Night
Pick a theme (like romance, action, or a favorite decade) and watch movies
that fit the theme. Create themed snacks or drinks to go along with it.
-Benefit: It's an easy way to bring variety to your date nights and gives you
a chance to relax and enjoy time together.

6. Plan a Board Game or Card Game Night
Choose a board game or a deck of cards and have a fun, competitive date night playing together.
-Benefit: Playing games can reduce stress, build communication, and bring out your playful sides, fostering a sense of fun.

7. Create a Mini At-Home Spa Night
Set up candles, play relaxing music, and take turns giving each other massages or facials.
-Benefit: Physical touch and relaxation help reduce stress and build intimacy, while giving you both time to unwind together.

8. Make a Bucket List Together
Sit down with your partner and create a bucket list of things you want to do together, from vacations to experiences at home.
-Benefit: Dreaming and planning for the future together keeps you aligned as a couple and gives you both something exciting to look forward to.

9. Have a Backyard Picnic
Lay out a blanket in the backyard, pack some snacks or dessert, and enjoy a romantic picnic under the stars.
-Benefit: Getting outside can create a new environment for bonding, and the novelty of a backyard picnic adds a special touch to the evening.

10. Plan a Dessert Date
Once the kids are in bed, prepare or order your favorite desserts and enjoy them together.
-Benefit: Indulging in a sweet treat together can create a relaxing and enjoyable experience, making the evening feel special.

11. Watch the Sunrise Together
Set your alarm early, make some coffee or tea, and sit outside or by a window to watch the sunrise.
-Benefit: Sharing quiet, peaceful moments at the start of the day brings a sense of calm and connection, while enjoying nature together.

12. Do a DIY Home Project Together
Pick a small home project or craft, like painting a room or building furniture, and work on it as a team.
-Benefit: Working together on a project builds teamwork, communication, and a sense of accomplishment when it's finished.

13. Have a Virtual Travel Night
Choose a destination you'd love to visit and recreate the experience at home with food, music, and maybe even a documentary about that place.
-Benefit: Exploring new cultures, even virtually, creates excitement and gives you a break from the everyday routine.

14. Write Love Notes to Each Other
Take some time to write short, meaningful notes or letters to each other and then exchange and read them together.
-Benefit: Expressing your feelings in writing helps deepen emotional intimacy and reminds you both of the love and appreciation you share.

15. Plan a 'No Technology' Night
Put away phones, tablets, and computers for the evening. Spend the time talking, playing games, or just enjoying each other's company.
-Benefit: Disconnecting from technology allows for undivided attention, deepening your emotional connection without distractions.

16. Read a Book Together
Pick a book you both want to read and either read it aloud to each other or read it separately and discuss as you go.
Benefit: Sharing a story or book can spark conversations, encourage thoughtful discussions, and give you a common interest.

17. Do a Puzzle Together
Work on a puzzle that you can spread out on a table and complete over a
few nights.
-Benefit: Puzzles provide a calming and collaborative activity, allowing you
to spend time together while engaging your minds.

18. Dance in the Living Room
Put on your favorite music, clear a space, and have an impromptu dance
party.
-Benefit: Dancing together releases endorphins, reduces stress, and lets
you both have fun, creating spontaneous moments of joy.

19. Plan Future Dates or Vacations
Even if you can't go out, take time to plan future date nights or vacations
you want to take together.
-Benefit: It keeps the excitement alive and gives you both something to look
forward to, strengthening your long-term connection.

20. Have a Candlelit Dinner
Set up a romantic dinner at home, with candles, soft music, and your
favorite meal.
-Benefit: A candlelit dinner feels intimate and special, creating a space for
meaningful conversation and connection.

My husband and I have made it a point to avoid using our phones when we're together unless we're looking something up together or taking pictures. It's a way to stay present, to be fully there in the moment. With life moving so fast, it's easy to get distracted, but we've learned that when we're intentional about putting our phones away, we connect on a much deeper level. It's about truly seeing each other and making the most of the time we have, which is precious when you're raising a family.

Finding someone to watch all the kids is rare, so we've had to get creative. We put the kids to bed at the same time every night, and that's when we get our alone time together. It's a sacred part of our day, helping us both wind down from the chaos. And on the weekends, if we wake up before the kids, we get those quiet morning moments too, sipping coffee and just enjoying each other's company. We value that time so much because it reminds us that even in the middle of parenting, we're still a team, still a couple with our own bond.

When we're with family, we make it a point to show affection—cuddling, holding hands, hugging. It's not just important for us, but it's something we want to normalize for our kids. I don't want them to think hugs are only for when someone is hurt or when we're leaving. I want them to see that affection can happen just because you love someone. It's a small but powerful way to model love for them, showing that connection is more than just words—it's the little acts of touch and care that matter.

Planning trips together has also become something we cherish. Not only does it give us something to look forward to, but it also helps us save money when we plan in advance, which reduces stress. Knowing we have something exciting on the horizon brings us closer, whether it's a weekend getaway or a bigger family vacation.

Whatever we do, we try to be fully present in those moments. Whether it's a quick hug, a quiet conversation after the kids are in bed, or dreaming about our next trip, we know how important it is to be there fully.

Open Communication Tips

1. Never Lie
Always be truthful, even when it's uncomfortable. Make honesty a habit in all conversations.
-Benefit: Builds trust and establishes a strong foundation for the relationship, reducing misunderstandings and resentment.

2. Never Keep Anything From Them
Be open about everything, whether it's small frustrations or big concerns. Keep your partner in the loop on what's happening in your life.
-Benefit: Transparency prevents surprises and builds emotional closeness, ensuring that both partners feel included in each other's lives.

3. Listen Without Judgment
Allow your partner to express their thoughts without interrupting or offering judgment. Focus on understanding their point of view.
-Benefit: Creates a safe space where both partners feel heard and accepted, strengthening emotional connection.

4. Don't Try to Fix Everything
Sometimes your partner just needs to vent or share their feelings. Resist the urge to offer solutions unless asked.
-Benefit: This shows empathy and respect for their feelings, helping them feel supported rather than dismissed or invalidated.

5. Focus on Listening Instead of Thinking About What to Say
Be fully present during conversations. Resist the urge to think of your response while they're still speaking.
-Benefit: Encourages active listening and deeper understanding, which leads to better communication and fewer misunderstandings.

6. Only Have Good Intentions
Approach every conversation with a positive mindset. Ensure your goal is
to strengthen the relationship, not to win an argument or prove a point.
-Benefit: Builds goodwill and creates a more loving and supportive
environment for both partners.

7. Don't Be Afraid to Apologize
When you're wrong, admit it and apologize sincerely. Don't let pride get in
the way of resolving conflicts.
-Benefit: Apologizing when necessary shows humility and respect, helping
to repair and strengthen your connection.

8. Know You're Not Always Right
Be open to the possibility that you might not have all the answers or may
have misunderstood something. Acknowledge when you've made a
mistake.
-Benefit: Being flexible and open-minded improves collaboration and helps
avoid unnecessary arguments.

9. Take Their Feelings Into Account
Consider your partner's emotions and perspective before speaking or
reacting. Validate their feelings even if you don't fully agree.
-Benefit: It fosters empathy and ensures that both partners feel respected
and understood, leading to healthier emotional exchanges.

10. Don't Cut Off Their Sentence
Let your partner finish their thought before responding. Resist the urge to
interrupt or cut them off.
-Benefit: Encourages full expression of thoughts and feelings, reducing
frustration and showing that you value what they have to say.

11. Show That You're Actively Listening
Use body language, such as nodding or making eye contact, to show
you're engaged. Reflect back what they've said to confirm understanding.
-Benefit: This shows that you care and are fully present in the conversation,
deepening your connection.

12. Ask Questions for Clarity
If something isn't clear, ask thoughtful questions to gain a better
understanding rather than assuming you know what they mean.
-Benefit: Helps avoid miscommunication and ensures you're both on the
same page.

13. Be Open About Your Own Feelings
Share your thoughts, concerns, and emotions with your partner regularly.
Don't bottle things up or wait for a breaking point.
-Benefit: Open sharing of feelings builds intimacy and trust, allowing both
partners to be more vulnerable and connected.

14. Create Regular Check-ins
Schedule time each week or month to talk about how you're feeling in the
relationship, how life is going, and any concerns.
-Benefit: Regular check-ins create space for open dialogue, helping prevent
resentment or issues from building up.

15. Don't Let Resentment Build
Address issues as they arise instead of letting them fester. Be open about
how you're feeling early on.
-Benefit: Tackling problems early prevents larger conflicts down the road
and promotes a healthier, happier relationship.

16. Avoid the Silent Treatment
When you're upset, express it constructively rather than giving your partner
the silent treatment or shutting down.
-Benefit: Open dialogue resolves issues faster and prevents emotional
distance, fostering a closer bond.

17. Be Honest About Your Needs
Don't expect your partner to read your mind. Clearly communicate what
you need from them emotionally, physically, and mentally.
-Benefit: Ensures that your needs are met and reduces misunderstandings,
leading to a more fulfilling relationship.

18. Respect Their Boundaries
If your partner needs space, alone time, or a moment to think, respect that.
Don't push for immediate resolutions.
-Benefit: Respecting boundaries promotes emotional safety and gives both
partners the time and space they need to process feelings.

19. Be Willing to Compromise
Understand that not every disagreement will end in your favor. Be open to
finding middle ground where both of you can be happy.
-Benefit: Compromise helps avoid conflict, fosters mutual respect, and
creates a balanced partnership where both voices are heard.

20. Speak Kindly, Even in Conflict
When addressing disagreements, use gentle, non-accusatory language.
Focus on expressing how you feel without blaming or attacking.
-Benefit: Kind communication minimizes defensiveness, leading to more
productive and respectful conversations.

I used to think that being completely honest with my partner was just a basic expectation, but now I realize how much freedom and peace it brings into our relationship. I never want to lie, especially to him, because there's no point in carrying the weight of secrets or guilt. It feels amazing to live without that burden, to truly be myself with him. My conscience is so clear, and that sense of relief is like nothing else.

One of the biggest lessons I've learned is to listen without judgment. If you judge your partner when they open up or vent to you, eventually they'll stop coming to you. They'll shut down, and the connection you share will start to fade. I used to think I had to fix everything, but sometimes, all he needed is someone to hear him, to let him unload what's weighing on his mind. I had to learn that it's okay for him to handle it on his own too; my role isn't always to jump in and solve things. Just being there, offering support, is often more important.

I try to do everything with good intentions, especially when it comes to our relationship. We used to argue over the dumbest things, only to realize later that it was all a misunderstanding or poor choice of words. What was meant as something positive would come out wrong, and before we knew it, we'd be arguing. But we've learned to step back, take a breath, and approach it differently. We look at each situation with the understanding that we love each other, that we wouldn't intentionally hurt one another. Now, instead of an argument, we have a conversation and usually end up realizing it was just a miscommunication.

Apologizing is no longer something we fear. Sure, it might take a little time to get there, but we both understand that pobody's nerfect. We've gotten into the habit of stepping away for a minute when things get tense, giving ourselves space to breathe and think. And most of the time, that's all it takes to clear our heads and remember what really matters. We don't let things ruin our day because at the end of it all, we love each other, and whatever went wrong isn't worth holding onto.

We've stopped going to bed angry too. I used to be guilty of the silent treatment, pulling the covers over my head like a cocoon and letting my frustration fester. It would build up inside until I'd explode over something small and insignificant. But I'm so grateful I've let go of that habit. Now, we talk things out, and we do it with open hearts and open minds.

One of the most important things we've learned is to compromise. We're lucky in that sense because we both care about making each other happy. When we face a disagreement, we work to find a balance. More often than not, the kids end up winning, but we always try to make sure everyone is content with the outcome. If something doesn't sit right with either of us, we make sure to cross it off the list. It's all about keeping each other's happiness in mind and finding resolutions that work for both of us.

Living this way has transformed our relationship, and I couldn't be more thankful for the peace and clarity we've found together.

Chapter 15
Is Your Family Complete?

Deciding if You Can Handle Another Baby

1. Emotional Readiness
Reflect on your current emotional state and whether you feel stable, happy, and mentally prepared to care for another child.
-Benefit: Ensuring emotional readiness can help you provide a loving, supportive environment for all your children.

2. Partner's Readiness
Discuss with your partner how they feel about having another child. Are both of you on the same page regarding this decision?
-Benefit: Mutual agreement strengthens your partnership and creates a balanced parenting dynamic.

3. Current Children's Needs
Evaluate how your existing children are doing. Are they in a phase that requires a lot of attention, or are they more independent?
-Benefit: Understanding your current family dynamic helps prevent overwhelm and ensures your kids get the attention they need.

4. Physical Health
Consult with your healthcare provider to determine if your body is physically ready for another pregnancy, especially if your last birth was recent.
-Benefit: Prioritizing your physical health ensures a smoother pregnancy and reduces potential complications.

5. Financial Stability
Review your financial situation, including the costs of healthcare, daycare, diapers, and other child-related expenses.
-Benefit: Financial stability helps reduce stress and ensures you can provide for your growing family comfortably.

6. Work-Life Balance
Consider your current job or career situation. Are you able to take time off
or adjust your schedule for a new baby?
-Benefit: A stable work-life balance allows you to spend quality time with
your children without sacrificing your professional life.

7. Support System
Assess the strength of your support system, including family, friends, and
childcare resources. Do you have people to rely on for help?
-Benefit: Having a reliable support system makes managing multiple
children much easier and reduces burnout.

8. Space in Your Home
Look at your current living space. Do you have enough room for another
child, or would you need to rearrange or move?
-Benefit: Ensuring adequate space helps reduce stress and keeps your
home comfortable and organized.

9. Your Energy Levels
Think about your current energy levels. Are you handling your daily routine
well, or are you already feeling exhausted with your current family setup?
-Benefit: Assessing your energy helps prevent physical and mental
burnout, ensuring you can meet the demands of another child.

10. Relationship Stability
Evaluate your relationship with your partner. Are you in a good place
emotionally and communicatively, or do you need to work through issues
first?
-Benefit: A strong relationship provides a stable environment for your
children and reduces stress during challenging parenting moments.

11. Impact on Current Routine
Consider how adding another baby will impact your family's routine. Are
you prepared for the disruption a new baby can bring?

-Benefit: Planning for routine changes ensures smoother transitions for everyone in the family.

12. Mental Health
Reflect on your mental health. Are you feeling mentally strong and capable, or are you currently struggling with stress, anxiety, or depression?
-Benefit: Mental well-being allows you to parent effectively and ensures you can meet the demands of another child without overwhelming yourself.

13. Timing
Think about the timing of having another child. Do you want your children close in age, or would you prefer to wait until your current children are older?
-Benefit: Thoughtful timing ensures you can balance the needs of each child while reducing stress for yourself and your partner.

14. Partner's Involvement
Discuss how involved your partner will be with the new baby. Are they able to share responsibilities equally?
-Benefit: Shared responsibilities create a balanced parenting dynamic, reducing the risk of one parent feeling overwhelmed.

15. Long-Term Goals
Consider your long-term goals as a family. Does adding another child align with your future plans, such as career growth, travel, or housing plans?
-Benefit: Aligning your decision with long-term goals helps ensure you're building the life you envision for your family.

16. Impact on Current Childcare
Assess how adding another baby will impact your current child care situation. Will you need more help, or can you handle the extra responsibility?
-Benefit: Understanding childcare needs ahead of time reduces stress and ensures each child gets adequate care.

17. Parenting Styles
Reflect on your current parenting style and how you handle discipline,
education, and emotional support. Can you manage another child with the
same approach, or will adjustments be needed?
-Benefit: Having a clear, consistent parenting style helps create a calm,
organized environment for your children.

18. Sleep
Consider how much sleep you're currently getting. Are you prepared for the
sleepless nights that come with a new baby?
-Benefit: Being realistic about sleep helps prevent exhaustion and allows
you to plan for periods of rest.

19. Desire for Another Child
Ask yourself if the desire for another child is coming from a deep, genuine
place, or if it's influenced by societal pressure or other factors.
-Benefit: Making this decision based on true desire ensures long-term
satisfaction with your family size.

20. Future Planning
Think about how another child fits into your family's future, including
education, vacations, and future financial needs.
-Benefit: Planning for the future gives you confidence that you're making
the

When our first set of babies were still toddlers, barely out of infancy, my husband sat me down one day and said something that completely threw me. He confessed that he wanted more kids. My first reaction? A mix of disbelief and exhaustion. Yeah, right, I thought. Both of our kids were still in diapers, teething, and every day felt like I was juggling just to keep everything together. How could we possibly handle more?

But because I love him, and I care about his feelings, I didn't shut it down. I simply said, "I'll think about it." And I really did. For months, I wrestled with the idea. My inner demons had a field day, filling me with doubt. You're barely managing now, they whispered. You're not good enough. You're already stretched thin.

Still, I couldn't shake it. I started imagining what it would be like to rearrange our house, to make space for more children, to adjust to an even busier life. But the real turning point wasn't about logistics or whether I could handle the chaos. It was about the future. Every time I thought about what our family might look like, I saw more. I saw a bigger, fuller family. And somehow, I just knew we would be okay.

I understood that things would get harder at times, but that didn't scare me. Instead, I realized I just needed to redefine what "hard" meant for me and grow into it. I had to grow as a person and as a mother. I needed to battle those voices in my head that kept telling me I wasn't good enough, and I needed to find strength I didn't know I had.

By confronting my negative self-talk, by finding and trusting myself, I became a better wife and mother. It wasn't easy, but I grew from it. And now, looking at our family, especially with our last two little ones, it blows my mind—and even hurts my heart a bit—to think that one decision, one conversation, could have changed everything.

If I had let fear or doubt win, these amazing, beautiful souls wouldn't be here. They light up our lives in ways I never imagined. They make me smile every single day. And I'm so grateful that I listened to my heart, found my strength, and said yes to the future I never knew I needed.

There's No "Right" Time to Have a Baby

1. Let Go of the Perfect Timeline
Stop waiting for the perfect moment when everything aligns
perfectly—career, finances, and life. Realize that life is unpredictable.
-Benefit: Reduces pressure and allows you to enjoy life's journey without
waiting for an elusive "ideal" moment.

2. Trust Your Instincts
Follow your inner feelings about whether or not you're ready for a baby
rather than adhering to external timelines.
-Benefit: Helps you make a decision based on your unique circumstances
and personal readiness, leading to greater fulfillment.

3. Focus on Health, Not Timing
Prioritize physical and emotional health when thinking about having a baby,
regardless of timing.
-Benefit: Ensures a better pregnancy and postpartum experience when
your focus is on well-being rather than arbitrary timing.

4. Embrace Life's Unpredictability
Accept that there will always be unexpected challenges in life, and having a
baby can bring joy amid them.
-Benefit: Reduces stress about needing everything to be "perfect" and
opens up to the joy of creating a family whenever it happens.

5. Don't Let Financial Concerns Paralyze You
While financial planning is important, recognize that no financial situation is
ever completely risk-free.
-Benefit: Frees you from waiting for an elusive financial milestone, allowing
you to embrace parenthood without indefinite delays.

6. Evaluate Current Family Dynamics
Assess your family's current needs and strengths to see if now is a good time for growth.
-Benefit: Helps you make a decision based on the present, not waiting for some "future" when life is perfect.

7. Know There's Never a 'Perfect' Job Scenario
If waiting for the "right" job or promotion is holding you back, consider that your career will continue to evolve, baby or not.
-Benefit: Allows you to move forward without compromising personal goals, making room for family and career growth.

8. Prioritize Relationships Over Timing
Focus on the strength and quality of your relationship with your partner rather than waiting for external circumstances to align.
-Benefit: A strong partnership offers support through any life stage, making parenting together more rewarding.

9. Stop Comparing Yourself to Others
Recognize that everyone's journey is unique, and comparing yourself to others' timelines doesn't benefit you.
-Benefit: Frees you from societal expectations and allows you to focus on what's right for your own family.

10. Recognize Personal Growth Happens Over Time
Understand that you don't need to have "everything figured out" before becoming a parent. Parenting is a journey of learning.
-Benefit: Alleviates the pressure of needing to be perfect and helps you grow into the role of a parent naturally.

11. Be Open to Unexpected Opportunities
Consider that life may present you with opportunities for family expansion in unexpected ways or times.
-Benefit: Keeps you flexible and adaptable to life's surprises, including a growing family.

12. Acknowledge the Biological Reality
Understand that while there's no perfect time, there are biological factors to consider regarding fertility.
-Benefit: Balances realistic considerations about fertility with an acceptance that there's never a fully ideal moment to start a family.

13. Focus on Emotional Preparedness
Shift the focus from external circumstances to whether you and your partner feel emotionally prepared for parenthood.
-Benefit: Strengthens your bond and builds a solid emotional foundation for family life.

14. Make Time for Connection
Before starting a family, focus on strengthening your relationship with your partner and nurturing your emotional connection.
-Benefit: Creates a strong, unified front for raising children together, no matter when they arrive.

15. Be Prepared for Change, Not Control
Instead of waiting for everything to be "in control," prepare yourself for the constant change that comes with having children.
-Benefit: Helps you embrace the unpredictability of life, knowing you'll adapt as circumstances shift.

16. Understand That Career Growth Can Coexist with Parenthood
Instead of viewing a baby as an interruption to your career, see it as an opportunity to grow in both areas of life.
-Benefit: Reduces fears that parenting will stall career progress and helps you see that growth can happen on multiple fronts.

17. Lean on Your Support System
Focus on the support available to you from family, friends, or community
when deciding if you're ready.
-Benefit: Knowing you have help enables you to take on parenthood
without needing everything to be perfect beforehand.

18. Don't Wait for Confidence—It Grows with Parenthood
Accept that you may not feel fully confident when deciding to have a baby
but trust that confidence grows with experience.
-Benefit: Encourages you to trust in your abilities and take the leap into
parenthood without needing to feel "ready" in every sense.

19. Focus on Small, Actionable Steps
Break down your concerns into smaller, manageable actions rather than
focusing on the big picture of parenthood.
-Benefit: Reduces overwhelm and shows that even small steps forward,
like researching or preparing, can make a big difference.

20. Celebrate the Present Moment
Shift your mindset from waiting for the "right" time to appreciating what you
have now and building from there.
-Benefit: Emphasizes the importance of living in the present, which creates
a positive and fulfilling atmosphere for both you and your future child.

Before my daughter was born, we tried for three long years. That's 36 times getting my period, 36 disappointments. We experienced early miscarriages, which left us heartbroken every time. We went to countless doctors, spent money on tests, treatments, and appointments, but nothing seemed to work. We had everything we thought we needed: jobs, healthcare, maternity leave, and a three-bedroom rental house that felt like it was waiting for a baby. But that baby just wouldn't come.

Eventually, we decided to focus on ourselves. We worked on our fitness and our mental health, trying to rebuild our spirits. We even started the process to foster-to-adopt, attending meetings, filling out stacks of paperwork, and preparing our home. I remember setting up the nursery in a Winnie the Pooh theme, just as I had always dreamed. But the reality was hard to accept: this baby we were preparing for would likely be temporary, a foster child we would care for until they went back to their biological family. It was a bittersweet moment—wanting so much to be parents but facing the idea that it might not be our own child.

One evening, after work, I came home to find my husband in that nursery, cuddling his childhood Pooh Bear. He looked so defeated, the saddest I had ever seen him. He wanted our own child—our own baby—to be in that crib. And in that moment, I didn't know what to say. I felt just as lost and broken, though I still had a sliver of hope left inside me.

A few days later, I decided to take a pregnancy test, not expecting much. But then, boom—pregnant. It felt like a miracle after all the waiting. I knew stress had been a huge factor, wreaking havoc on my body, so I made the decision to step back from a lot of things. That choice upset some people, but I didn't explain much. We kept the pregnancy a secret, knowing we needed to protect it, to guard it fiercely after everything we had been through. Good thing we did because the pregnancy was rough. But looking back now, seeing my daughter today, I realize the timing was perfect. She came exactly when she was meant to.

After she was born, I was on my way to get birth control, ready to plan our family's next step. I was sitting in the parking lot when my husband called. He simply said, "I really don't want you to get it." And I felt instant relief, responding, "Me too." We both thought, after three years of trying, it would probably take at least a year for another baby to come. But two months later—boom—pregnant again.

At that time, we weren't as "ready" as we were before. We had moved into a one-bedroom apartment, with no yard, and I wasn't working. We were freaking out, our minds racing with worries. But deep down, we knew we would figure it out, even if we didn't have all the answers yet. And when our second baby arrived, it was the biggest blessing. We loved how close in age they were, and it was so special that they would grow up together, side by side.

We loved it so much that we did it on purpose the next time, bringing another set of babies into the world. By the time they came, we had our house and land, ready to embrace the chaos of a bigger family. Looking back, I realize you're never truly "ready" for what life throws at you—you just get ready. And somehow, you find your way, step by step, one baby at a time.

Imagining the Future of Your Family

1. Define Your Family Values
Sit down with your partner and discuss the core values you want to instill in
your family, such as kindness, respect, and responsibility.
-Benefit: Establishing values creates a strong foundation that will guide
your family's decisions and interactions in the future.

2. Visualize Long-Term Goals
Think about where you'd like to see your family in 5, 10, or 20 years. This
could include family size, career balance, or lifestyle changes.
-Benefit: Provides a sense of direction and purpose, ensuring that your
decisions today align with your long-term vision.

3. Consider Financial Planning
Assess your current financial situation and start planning for future
expenses like education, housing, and retirement.
-Benefit: Reduces financial stress down the line and ensures that you are
prepared for both expected and unexpected costs.

4. Plan for Education and Learning
Discuss how you want to approach your children's education—whether
homeschooling, public school, or alternative methods.
-Benefit: Early planning allows you to adapt your approach to education
based on each child's individual needs, ensuring they thrive academically
and personally.

5. Prioritize Emotional Growth
Focus on raising emotionally intelligent children by teaching them how to
express their feelings, handle stress, and develop empathy.
-Benefit: Prepares your children for healthy relationships and emotional
resilience throughout life.

6. Create Family Traditions
Establish meaningful family traditions, such as holiday celebrations, weekly family dinners, or yearly vacations.
-Benefit: Traditions build lasting memories, create a sense of belonging, and strengthen family bonds.

7. Think About Physical and Mental Health
Prioritize healthy habits for your family, such as balanced nutrition, regular exercise, and mental health check-ins.
-Benefit: Ensures that your family remains physically and mentally strong, laying the groundwork for a healthier future.

8. Plan for Time Together and Apart
Make time for both family activities and individual pursuits. Encourage everyone in the family to follow their own passions.
-Benefit: Strengthens both family unity and personal growth by allowing space for connection and independence.

9. Set Up a Safety Net
Create a plan for emergencies, such as medical issues, financial downturns, or natural disasters.
-Benefit: Provides peace of mind knowing that you're prepared for the unexpected, keeping your family safe and secure.

10. Focus on the Environment You Want to Create
Envision the type of home environment you want to cultivate, whether it's warm and cozy, structured and orderly, or creative and flexible.
-Benefit: Creating a nurturing home environment positively impacts your family's overall well-being and daily interactions.

11. Think About Aging and Elder Care
Discuss with your partner how you want to handle aging parents or grandparents, whether it's in-home care, assisted living, or other options.
-Benefit: Preparing for elder care ensures smoother transitions and avoids last-minute decisions during a stressful time.

12. Imagine How to Balance Work and Family Life
Think about your ideal balance between work and family. Consider career flexibility, remote work, or reducing work hours if necessary.
-Benefit: Ensures that your family's needs are met without sacrificing personal career goals, leading to better work-life harmony.

13. Consider How to Handle Family Challenges
Prepare for potential challenges, such as sibling rivalry, academic struggles, or health issues, and how you might address them together.
-Benefit: Proactively considering challenges fosters resilience and problem-solving skills within the family.

14. Think About Family Legacy
Reflect on the legacy you want to leave behind, whether it's through traditions, values, financial security, or personal stories.
-Benefit: Building a family legacy instills a sense of pride and continuity, helping future generations feel connected to their roots.

15. Plan for Personal Growth as Parents
Set goals for how you want to grow as parents, such as improving patience, communication, or parenting strategies.
-Benefit: Focusing on self-improvement strengthens your role as a parent and enhances the overall family dynamic.

16. Discuss Family Expansion
Regularly revisit discussions about whether or when to expand your family, factoring in your current circumstances and future goals.
-Benefit: Ongoing dialogue ensures that both partners are aligned on family size and timing, reducing tension or misunderstandings.

17. Think About Future Family Milestones
Consider what future milestones—such as first days of school, graduations,
or weddings—you'll want to celebrate as a family.
-Benefit: Anticipating these moments fosters excitement and planning,
making it easier to be present and engaged when they happen.

18. Plan for Conflict Resolution
Establish guidelines for resolving family conflicts, whether it's between
partners or children. Focus on healthy communication and compromise.
-Benefit: Reduces stress and creates a culture of understanding and
respect, ensuring that disagreements don't spiral into long-term issues.

19. Think About Travel and Exploration
Plan for future family adventures, whether it's local weekend trips or
international vacations.
-Benefit: Traveling together strengthens bonds, broadens horizons, and
creates cherished family memories.

20. Foster Lifelong Learning
Encourage lifelong learning within your family, whether through hobbies,
educational pursuits, or skills development.
-Benefit: Promotes curiosity, creativity, and personal growth, ensuring that
each family member continues to evolve and thrive.

I was born with a bad heart, so I always knew that having children would be hard on my body. But it was a priority for me to have kids before I turned 30. My husband had his own reasons—he was adopted by older parents, and his biggest fear was that his children might not remember them. Together, we had a vision for our family. We wanted to spend our later years traveling, exploring the world together, something that becomes harder when you're still raising young children. Everything pointed to one thing: we needed to have our children as soon as possible.

We knew it wouldn't be easy. It would put a strain on my heart, and the challenges of raising kids back-to-back were clear. But it was something we both believed was worth it. Our children, and the life we imagined with them, outweighed any difficulties we might face along the way.

We also wanted our children to have each other. I'd watched my stepson grow up all alone for his first five years, and it was heartbreaking at times. We didn't want that for our future kids—we wanted them to have a built-in buddy, someone to grow up alongside. It was important to us that they had siblings close in age, so they could experience childhood together, create memories they'd share forever, and be there for eachother when we are gone.

Another important decision we made was that I would stay home with the kids. We didn't want someone else raising them or witnessing their milestones while we were away at work. It wasn't just about being present; it was about being the ones guiding their growth and sharing in those first steps, first words, and everything in between. Financially, it made sense for us, but more than that, it felt right for our family. We wanted to build traditions and routines together, creating a strong foundation for our kids to thrive in.

As we started our family, those early traditions we built were not only a great experience—they also showed us how far we've come. Looking back, I see that every struggle and challenge was part of a bigger plan. Our family is stronger because of it, and it gives me so much hope for the future. We did what we set out to do, and while life isn't always easy, we're proud of the life we've built for our children and the memories we're making along the way.

Trusting Your Instincts and Vision for Your Family

1. Acknowledge Your Unique Parenting Style
Recognize that your parenting style is shaped by your experiences and values, and it may look different from others'.
-Benefit: Embracing your uniqueness reduces the pressure to conform and builds confidence in your approach.

2. Listen to Your Gut Feelings
Pay attention to the feelings you get when making decisions about your family. If something feels wrong or right, take note.
-Benefit: Trusting your gut can help you make quicker and more aligned decisions, especially in high-pressure moments.

3. Reflect on Past Successes
Look back at situations where your instincts led to positive outcomes for your family.
-Benefit: Reflecting on past successes boosts confidence and reassures you that your instincts have value.

4. Filter Out Outside Noise
Limit how much advice you take from others, especially unsolicited advice. Focus on what works best for your family.
-Benefit: Reducing external influence helps you stay true to your vision and lowers stress from conflicting opinions.

5. Stay Educated but Selective
Research parenting tips and expert advice, but adapt them to suit your family's unique dynamics.
-Benefit: Staying informed ensures you're making educated decisions while still honoring your instincts.

6. Practice Self-Reflection
Regularly take time to reflect on your parenting decisions and how they align with your overall vision for your family.
-Benefit: Self-reflection fosters personal growth and clarity, making it easier to trust your instincts moving forward.

7. Communicate with Your Partner
Discuss your family vision with your partner to ensure you're both on the same page and can support each other's instincts.
-Benefit: Open communication strengthens trust between partners and allows for shared decision-making based on instincts.

8. Respect Your Children's Individuality
Trust your instincts to guide each child in their unique needs and personality, rather than following a one-size-fits-all approach.
-Benefit: Fosters a deeper connection with each child and ensures that they feel understood and valued.

9. Learn to Say No
If something doesn't align with your vision or doesn't feel right, trust yourself to say no—even to well-meaning suggestions from others.
-Benefit: Saying no when needed establishes boundaries and keeps your family on track with its goals and values.

10. Visualize Your Family's Future
Take time to imagine what you want your family's future to look like. What values, routines, or achievements are important to you?
-Benefit: Visualization helps clarify your long-term vision, making it easier to trust the path you're taking today.

11. Give Yourself Permission to Make Mistakes
Understand that mistakes are a natural part of parenting. Trust that you'll learn and grow from each experience.
-Benefit: Relieves pressure and helps you move forward without fear, strengthening your belief in your instincts.

12. Limit Comparisons
Avoid comparing your family or parenting style to others, whether in real life
or on social media.
-Benefit: Prevents feelings of inadequacy and ensures that you stay true to
your unique family vision.

13. Act on Your First Reaction
When making decisions, try following your first instinct before overthinking
or second-guessing.
-Benefit: Acting on your first reaction can save time and prevent decision
fatigue, especially when dealing with daily challenges.

14. Celebrate Small Wins
Acknowledge and celebrate the small victories that come from following
your instincts, whether it's handling a tantrum or navigating a family
challenge.
-Benefit: Celebrating small wins reinforces that your instincts are guiding
you in the right direction.

15. Stay Flexible
While trusting your instincts, remain open to adjusting your vision when
circumstances change or new information arises.
-Benefit: Flexibility allows you to adapt while still staying grounded in your
overall vision for the family.

16. Create a Family Vision Board
Create a vision board with your partner that represents your family goals
and values. Include visuals that inspire you.
-Benefit: A visual reminder of your family's goals keeps you focused and
reinforces your instincts when making decisions.

17. Trust Your Bond with Your Children
Pay attention to the emotional bond you have with your children, and let
that connection guide your parenting decisions.
-Benefit: A strong parent-child bond deepens trust in your instincts,
especially when making decisions that directly affect your children.

18. Practice Patience
Trusting your instincts doesn't always lead to immediate results. Practice
patience and give your decisions time to unfold.
-Benefit: Patience fosters a sense of calm and reduces frustration, making
it easier to follow through on your instincts.

19. Trust Your Parenting Experience
Rely on the lessons and experiences you've gained from parenting each of
your children, knowing that these shape your instincts.
-Benefit: Drawing from experience increases your confidence and helps
you trust that your past decisions have prepared you for future ones.

20. Make Space for Self-Care
Ensure that you're taking care of yourself physically and emotionally, as a
healthy mindset strengthens your ability to trust your instincts.
-Benefit: Self-care helps you stay balanced and resilient, making it easier to
act on your instincts with clarity and confidence.

Before I had kids, I thought I had a clear outline for how I was going to raise mine. I'd worked with children for years, helped raise my siblings, and had already been a stepmom. I figured that experience would make it easier, that I'd be fully prepared when my time came. But reality was different. The minute I had my own babies, all those plans went out the window.

Don't get me wrong—my past experience did help, but I quickly realized I had to discover my own parenting style. It wasn't about following a script or mimicking what I'd seen. It was about figuring out what worked for my kids, taking the good from my past and leaving the rest behind. There were things I thought I'd do for sure, but when the time came, I realized they just weren't for me. And that's okay. Everyone has their own way of raising kids, and there's nothing wrong if others believe in things that didn't work for me.

Along the way, I also had to block out all the outside noise. There were so many opinions—from family, friends, even strangers in the store. Some people couldn't believe we were having kids at all, and most couldn't wrap their heads around the idea of four under five. I can't walk into a store without at least five people commenting on how many kids I have. I get it—I used to be the one saying, "Wow, that's a lot of kids." Now, I'm on the other side of that conversation. But to us, it's beautiful. Our family is exactly what it's meant to be, and I wouldn't change a thing.

In the end, there are so many parenting approaches, so many judgmental eyes out there. But what I've learned is that if you raise your kids with their best interests in mind, with an open heart and an open mind, and if you're always willing to learn and grow as a parent, you're going to be okay. There's no perfect way to parent. It's about doing your best, trusting your instincts, and loving your kids the way only you can.

This book is dedicated to my children, my siblings and to all the mothers out there looking for guidance. May this book help you in any way possible and unconditional love guide you.